KU-546-540

AN ILLUSTRATED COLOUR TEXT

General
Practice
Medicine

ts
als wor

you are accept

eturned to the BMA

until the date stamped

items can be recalled after one

g by post, please ensure that you obtain
om the Post Office; oth   you will be li

19 AUG 200

25/20

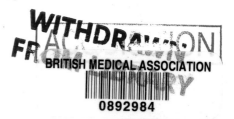

WITHDRAWN
FROM LIBRARY
BRITISH MEDICAL ASSOCIATION

0892984

Commissioning Editor: Ellen Green
Project Development Manager: Lynn Watt, Jim Killgore
Project Manager: Frances Affleck
Designer: Sarah Russell
Illustration Manager: Bruce Hogarth

AN ILLUSTRATED COLOUR TEXT

General Practice Medicine

Ross J. Taylor MB, ChB, MD, FRCPE, FRCGP, DCH

Department of General Practice and Primary Care
Forresterhill Health Centre
Aberdeen, UK

Brian R. McAvoy MB, ChB, MD, FRACGP, FRNZCGP, FRCGP, FRCP, FAChAM, BSc

Deputy Director
National Cancer Control Initiative
Adjunct and Honorary Professor of General Practice
Universities of Melbourne, Monash and Queensland, Australia

Tom O'Dowd MB, Bch, MA, MD, MICGP, FRCGP

Professor of General Practice Medicine
University of Dublin
Trinity College
Dublin, Ireland

Illustrated by Graham Chambers

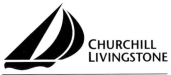

CHURCHILL
LIVINGSTONE

EDINBURGH   LONDON   NEW YORK   PHILADELPHIA   ST LOUIS   SYDNEY   TORONTO   2003

CHURCHILL LIVINGSTONE
An imprint of Elsevier Science Limited

First published 2003

ISBN 0443 06045 2

British Library Cataloguing in Publication Data
A catalogue record for this book is available from the British Library

Library of Congress Cataloging in Publication Data
A catalog record for this book is available from the Library of Congress

Note
Medical knowledge is constantly changing. As new information becomes
available, changes in treatment, procedures, equipment and the use of
drugs become necessary. The authors and the publishers have taken care
to ensure that the information given in this text is accurate and up to date.
However, readers are strongly advised to confirm that the information,
especially with regard to drug usage, complies with the latest legislation
and standards of practice.

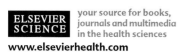

your source for books,
journals and multimedia
in the health sciences

www.elsevierhealth.com

The
publisher's
policy is to use
**paper manufactured
from sustainable forests**

Printed in Spain

PREFACE

One of the major recent changes in medical education is the greater use of general practice to provide opportunities for the clinical education of students outside the hospital environment. This is partly because of a realisation that hospital based education cannot by itself provide comprehensive clinical experience, and partly because of the increasing logistical difficulties of basing medical education entirely on hospitals at a time when, for example, care is being transferred from secondary to primary care, hospital stays are generally shorter and most chronic diseases (e.g. asthma, ischaemic heart disease, arthritis) are mainly dealt with by general practitioners. The General Medical Council also recommends early exposure of students to patients and an integration of clinical and pre-clinical phases. Many schools see this as a natural place for learning in general practice and it is likely that most will have such a scheme in addition to, or instead of, senior clinical attachments to general practices.

The purpose of this textbook is to help the student make the most out of the experience of early clinical attachment to general practices, however this is arranged. The book should:

- familiarise the student with the context of general practice, i.e. the major ways in which it is different from hospital based care
- give the student a simple, general overview of clinical work in general practice
- give the student a framework for learning from general practice and alert him/her to relevant opportunities for learning, giving examples
- fill in gaps in clinical knowledge which are not adequately covered by hospital based clinical textbooks.

Rather than supplanting existing textbooks, this book is designed to be used in conjunction with other texts, particularly those from the ICT (Illustrated Colour Text) series. It follows the successful format of this series, with an emphasis on integrated text/illustration, generally following the formula of one topic per double page spread. In selecting and arranging content the editors have rigorously excluded irrelevance and pursued authoritative material based as far as possible on the most recent evidence. The over-riding aim is to illustrate important general principles about clinical method (in its broadest sense) in the context of general practice. The book is therefore neither comprehensive nor detailed in its description of clinical conditions, this being the purpose of other associated texts.

R. J.T.
B.R.M.
T.O'D

ACKNOWLEDGEMENTS

The authors would like to thank the following for their contribution to this book:

Dr Fiona Bradley
Lecturer in General Practice
University of Dublin
Trinity College
Dublin, Ireland
(Fiona died on 25 November 2002 aged 41 years)
Evidence-based medicine

Professor Patrick Pietroni
Regional Education Support Unit
St Charles Hospital
London, UK
Complementary and alternative medicine

Dr Peter Rose
Millstone Surgery
Wallingford, UK
Genetics in primary care

Dr Susan Smith
Lecturer in General Practice
University of Dublin
Trinity College
Dublin, Ireland
Common mental health problems
Common gastrointestinal disorders

Dr Edwin van Teijlingen
Co-ordinator MSc Health Services and Public Health Research,
Department of Public Health and Dugald Baird Centre for Research on Women's Health
Department of Public Health
Aberdeen, UK
Changes in society

Thanks are also due to the team at Elsevier, including Lynn Watt, Project Development Manager.

R. J.T.
B.R.M.
T.O'D

CONTENTS

COMMON CHRONIC HEALTH PROBLEMS

SPECIAL TOPICS

APPENDICES

INDEX

Importance and relevance of primary health care

Primary health care (PHC) as a concept was officially launched in 1978 at a World Health Organization (WHO)/UNICEF conference in Alma-Ata, in the former Soviet Union, at which some 150 governments were represented. The Alma-Ata Declaration (World Health Organization 1978) defined PHC as follows:

Primary health care is essential health care based on practical, scientifically sound and socially acceptable methods and technology made universally accessible to individuals and families in the community through their participation and at a cost that the community and country can afford to maintain at every stage of their development in the spirit of self-reliance and self-determination. It forms an integral part both of the country's health system, of which it is the central function and main focus, and of the overall social and economic development of the community. It is the first level of contact of individuals, the family and community with the national health system bringing health care as close as possible to where people live and work, and constitutes the first element of a continuing health care process.

The Alma-Ata Declaration identified 10 activities as the basic elements of PHC (Table 1); as can be seen, general practice is only one component of this broader definition (Box 1). The Declaration contains important socio-political implications that address not only treating disease, but also ensuring fair access to a positive state of well-being for all citizens. It recognises the social, economic and environmental determinants of health and promotes the importance of community

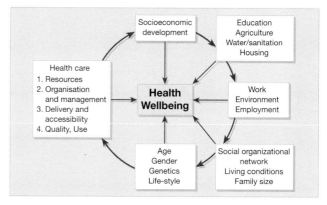

Fig. 1 **Determinants of health.** Adapted from Tarimo and Webster (1994).

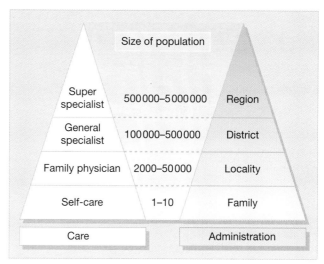

Fig. 2 **Levels of care and administration.** Source: Fry and Sandler (1993).

participation. It also acknowledges that improvements in health result mainly from activities outside the health sector (Fig. 1).

Fry and Sandler (1993) have described four-levels of care and administration in all health-care systems that relate to population size and the nature of disease and other problems at each level (Fig. 2). Primary care provides the first level of professional care within a locality or community, occupying the interface between self-care and hospital-based secondary (general specialist) and tertiary (superspecialist) care.

PHC can be viewed in four ways (Vuori 1986):

1. *as a set of activities*: as outlined in the Alma-Ata Declaration (Table 1);
2. *as a level of care*: PHC being that part of the care system which people contact first when they have a health problem;
3. *as a strategy for organising health services*: defined as accessible care, relevant to the needs of the population, functionally integrated, based on community participation, cost-effective and characterised by collaboration between all sectors of society. This may also require a re-orientation of health personnel and resources from tertiary and secondary to primary health care.
4. *as a philosophy that should permeate the entire health-care system*: the essence of the PHC movement. A

Box 1 Defining primary health care

- Value driven: dignity, equity, solidarity and ethics
- Protects and promotes health
- Centred on people but allowing self reliance
- Focus is quality including cost effectiveness
- Sustainable finances, allowing universal coverage and equitable access

Source: Ljubljana Charter, WHO, adopted by EU (1996)

Table 1 Basic elements of primary health care

- Health education
- Identifying and controlling prevailing health problems
- Food supply and proper nutrition
- Provision of safe water and basic sanitation
- Maternal and child health care, including family planning
- Immunisation
- Prevention and control of endemic disease
- Appropriate treatment of common diseases and injuries
- Promotion of mental health
- Provision of essential drugs

Source: Tarima and Webster (1978)

country can claim to practise PHC only if its entire health-care system is characterised by social justice and equality, international solidarity, self-responsibility and an acceptance of the broad definition of health.

The role of primary health care

The primary care physician has a number of functions (World Health Organization 1971):

- to provide continuous and comprehensive care
- to refer to specialists and/or hospital services
- to co-ordinate health services for the patient
- to guide the patient within the network of social welfare and public health services
- to provide the best possible health and social services in the light of economic considerations.

In the UK primary care physicians are known as general practitioners (Box 2). The term 'gatekeeper' has been used to describe the GP's role in determining patients' access to specialist services.

In order to fulfil these functions, the doctor requires four skills specific to general practice (McWhinney 1997):

1. skills to solve undifferentiated problems in the context of a continuing personal relationship with individuals and families
2. preventive skills – the identification of risks and early departure from normality in patients who are known to the doctor
3. therapeutic skills – the use of the doctor – patient relationship to maximise the effectiveness of all kinds of therapy
4. Resource management skills – the deployment of the resources of the community and the health care system for the benefit of patients.

As teaching and research have become more mainstream activities within PHC, doctors have recently had to acquire skills in these areas too.

The benefits of primary health care

Health service reforms in UK and around the world are moving towards primary care-centred services. The available evidence broadly supports this shift, although it also indicates the limits of substitution for secondary care. Starfield (1992) reviewed primary care in 11 Western nations, with the following conclusions:

Box 2 Definition of a general practitioner

- Provides personal, primary and continuing medical care to individuals and families
- Makes an initial decision on every problem presented
- Consults with specialists when appropriate
- Intervenes to promote health
- Clinical decisions influenced by prior probability of disease
- Has an advocacy role for the patient
- Specific responsibility for the health of the community

Sources: Royal College of General Practitioners 1992; WONCA Europe 2002

Box 3 Characteristics of general practice and primary health care

General practice	**Primary health care**
Focus is illness:	Focus is local communities:
■ Individuals and families	1. Local communities using local knowledge
■ First contact	2. Concerned about determinants of health
■ Local and accessible	■ Socio-economic
■ Small scale efficiency	■ Environmental
■ Tolerates uncertainty	3. Empowers communities to control/influence determinants of health
The three Cs: continuity, coordination, continuing care	4. Education and prevention are key pieces

---

- A higher primary care orientation is likely to produce better health for a population at a lower cost.
- Primary care is not necessarily synonymous with managed care (which restricts medical choice in terms of investigation, referral and treatment).
- The total health-care expenditure is generally higher in countries where health-care systems are left to the vagaries of market forces.
- Free market systems appear to have higher inpatient costs per capita and a higher per capita expenditure on medication.
- The restriction of specialists to hospitals and their payment by salary are generally associated with a better systems performance for the population as a whole.
- The regulation of the location of physicians and their equitable distribution across the population are generally associated with better health system performance.

The process that Starfield sees giving PHC its strengths is identified as

front-line, ongoing care that is comprehensive and coordinated. Further details are given on pages 10 and 11.

Other international studies have found associations between availability of PHC and health outcomes (including reduced hospital use), patient satisfaction and reduced health-care costs.

There is also evidence of positive benefits from shared care (between GPs and hospital specialists) for patients with asthma; hypertension; childhood cancers. The evidence for the cost-effectiveness of the primary care management of diabetes mellitus is, however, ambiguous, and there is some evidence that although patients' satisfaction and knowledge of their condition might be better, the level of control is poorer than with hospital management.

Although much of the political interest in PHC around the world has been driven by cost-containment agendas, primary care-centred services are not always cheaper than hospital-based services.

Primary care

- Primary health care can be seen as a set of activities, a level of care, a strategy for organising health services and a philosophy that should permeate the entire health care system.
- General practitioners have a key role as 'gatekeepers' in determining patients' access to specialist services.
- Primary health care is front-line, ongoing care which is comprehensive and coordinated.
- Health care systems with a higher primary care orientation tend to produce better health of a population at lower costs.

Overview and philosophy of generalist practice

General practice medicine is clinical medicine practised in the community, and at its core lies the consultation between doctor and patient. Sir James Spence (1960) described the consultation as follows:

The essential unit of medical practice is the occasion when, in the intimacy of the consulting room or sick room, a person who is ill or believes himself to be ill, seeks the advice of a doctor whom he trusts. This is a consultation and all else in the practice of medicine derives from it. The purpose of the consultation is that the doctor, having gathered his evidence, shall give explanation and advice.

The term 'general practitioner' came into use only at the beginning of the 19th century, and this doctor's appearance disturbed the long-existing stability in the provision of medical care in Britain. The respective territories of the learned physician, the craftsman surgeon and the tradesman apothecary had previously been well demarcated and fiercely guarded. The Medical Act of 1858 established a common course of training for all doctors. The discipline of general practice in Britain developed through the 19th century and into the 20th, strengthened by the implementation of Lloyd George's National Insurance Act in 1911 and the introduction of the National Health Service in 1948.

Definitions

A number of different terms are used around the world to describe the community-based clinical generalist doctor – GP, family physician, primary care physician or practitioner, family doctor. Similarly, there are several definitions, ranging from the simple – a doctor who provides personal, primary and continuing medical care to individuals, families and a practice population, irrespective of age, sex or illness – to more complex ones incorporating detailed job descriptions (see Box 1, p. 3).

Although the health system varies considerably between countries, the clinical generalist is an essential feature of an efficient and effective health service.

Differences between GPs and specialists

Over the past 30 years or so, there has been a trend towards increasing specialisation, fuelled by the burgeoning growth of technology and bioscientific discoveries. Paradoxically, the increasing sophistication and complexity of hospital-based specialist medicine has highlighted the need for high-quality clinical generalists in the community. The community-based generalist and the hospital specialist complement each other, but differ in their professional roles and attitudes, and the structure and content of their practice (Table 1). The role of the specialist is to reduce uncertainty, explore possibility and minimise error. The role of the GP is to accept uncertainty, explore probability and marginalise danger (Marinker 1990). Generalists do not have less knowledge or skill than specialists but use their different knowledge and skills in a different way. Good primary health care will need to build on the strengths of the clinical generalist and value breadth of knowledge as much as depth, and skills in listening and empathy as much as those of high-tech intervention.

Importance of clinical generalist

The medical generalist who is specifically trained to work in primary care has the breadth of training to cope flexibly with a wide range of conditions and the added value of relying more on clinically attuned ears and eyes than on expensive technology (Feinstein 1983). The clinical generalist is now viewed as an essential component of many Western nations' front-line services, for the following reasons (Royal College of General Practitioners 1996):

- The problems that people present to formal health services are undifferentiated in nature.
- The clinical epidemiology of front-line care is different from that of the more selected populations with which specialists deal. An understanding of front-line clinical probabilities and risk management is a prerequisite for the primary (generalist) physician's ability to tolerate clinical uncertainty and to use time rather than inappropriate expensive investigations.
- The clinical generalist will have the opportunity to value and utilise the continuing, longitudinal relationship

| Table 1 **Difference between general practice and hospital** | |
General practice–practitioner	Hospital–specialist
Structure	
Cares for a small registered population (2000)	Cares for a larger unregistered population (250 000+)
Patients registered with an individual doctor	No registration system
Patients have direct access	Access usually via GP
Situated close to patient's home	Situated far from most patients' homes
Huge variability between practices (e.g. age, social class of patients, geographical distribution)	Hospitals exhibit far less variability
Function	
Responsibility for *all* health care for patients	Responsibility for specialty-related *medical* care
Responsibility for all presenting problems irrespective of age, sex or morbidity	Responsible for specialty-related problems only: restricted by age (e.g. paediatrics) or sex (obstetrics and gynaecology)
Presented with undifferentiated problems/diseases	Presented with more organised disease
Deals with common diseases and social problems	Deals mainly with rare diseases or atypical versions of common diseases
Makes infrequent and highly selective use of 'high technology'	Makes frequent and less selective use of 'high technology'
Continuing responsibility for patients	Episodic responsibility for patients
Repeated opportunities for anticipatory care	Fewer opportunities for anticipatory care
Attitudes	
'Whole person' oriented: uses 'triple diagnosis'	Disease oriented: usually either physical or psychological
Prepared to use time as diagnostic tool (nice to know)	Little use of time as a diagnostic tool (need to know)
Importance of doctor–patient relationship and its uses are recognised and valued	Doctor–patient relationship less well demonstrated or used
If no cure, recognises the need for continuing care and support	If there is no cure, the patient is often discharged
Patient's viewpoint and autonomy recognised	Less recognition of patient's viewpoint and autonomy

Source: Fraser (1999)

with many patients. A professional who is able to match appropriate services against the needs of the individual has the potential to protect the public from excessive or insufficient intervention.

■ A separation of primary clinical assessment from decisions about who can receive very expensive technical interventions is desirable if members of the public are to feel that there is fairness and equity in their health care.

Context and content of general practice

The GP practises clinical medicine in a very different setting and context from those of the hospital specialist. Problems are often undifferentiated, illness is much more common than disease, and consequently the content of clinical practice is very different from that encountered in hospital. The most common cause of chest pain in patients presenting to hospital is, for example, cardiac in origin, whereas musculoskeletal disorders are the commonest cause of chest pain presenting in general practice.

Moreover, only 25% of patients who experience symptoms decide to cross the threshold between self-care and professional care by consulting a GP, and of those, only 10% are subsequently referred to hospital (Fig. 1). Consequently, 90% of episodes of illness presenting to the GP are managed entirely within primary care. Some symptoms are more likely to lead to a consultation than others (Table 2).

Sixty per cent of consultations are for minor self-limiting problems (e.g. upper respiratory tract infections or gastrointestinal upsets), 25% for chronic non-curable conditions (e.g.

Table 2 **Likelihood of symptoms leading to consultation**	
Symptoms	**Ratio of symptom episodes to consultation**
Changes in energy	456:1
Headache	184:1
Disturbance of gastric function	109:1
Backache	52:1
Pain in lower limb	49:1
Emotional/psychological	46:1
Abdominal pain	29:1
Disturbance of menstruation	20:1
Sore throat	18:1
Pain in chest	14:1

Source: Fraser (1999)

Table 2 **Reasons for patients visiting their GP, England and Wales, 1991/92 (rates per 10 000 person years at risk)**	
Acute upper respiratory infections	772
Acute bronchitis and bronchitis	719
Asthma	425
Disorders of the conjunctivae	415
Essential hypertension	412
Disorders of the external ear	409
Acute pharyngitis	409
Acute tonsillitis	407
Ill-defined intestinal infections	394
Other and unspecified disorders of the back	372

Source: Office of Population Censuses and Surveys (1995) Reproduced with permission from Morbidity Statistics from General Practice, National Statistics © Crown Copyright 2000

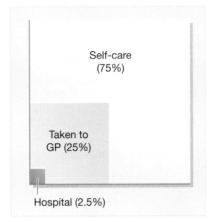

Fig. 1 **Levels of care of symptoms.**
Source: Fraser (1999)

hypertension or diabetes) and 15% for acute, major, life-threatening conditions (e.g. myocardial infarction or acute appendicitis).

The most common reason for patients consulting their doctor is for respiratory problems (31% of all consultations), followed by disorders of the nervous system (17%), musculoskeletal problems (15%) and skin disorders (15%), injury and poisoning (14%) and infectious or parasitic diseases (14%) (Office of Population Censuses and Surveys 1995). The reasons patients give for visiting their GP are shown in Table 2.

The broad range of skills required to fulfil the generalist role has been well described by Fraser (1999):

The general practitioner, therefore, particularly needs to develop skills as a primary assessor of problems in a situation where multiple problems are often presented in a single consultation, where there are many symptoms but few clinical signs, and where there is frequently a complex mix of physical, social and psychological factors. In particular he needs to develop the ability to be appropriately selective in history taking, in performing physical examinations and in use of investigative facilities. He also needs to tailor his approach to suit the individual patient.

For an example of a typical morning's surgery, please see Appendix 2, page 101.

> *Generalist practice*
>
> ■ Generalists and specialists require different knowledge, skills and attitudes but are complementary in their roles.
>
> ■ The GP is committed to the person rather than to a particular body of knowledge, a group of diseases or special techniques (McWhinney 1997)
>
> ■ A GP provides personal, primary and continuing care to individuals, families and a practice population.
>
> ■ The spectrum of problems presenting in general practice is very different from that seen in hospital.
>
> ■ The GP must combine the scientific and humanitarian approach to medical practice, providing holistic care to patients.

Models of health care

Caring for patients is attending to particulars, not dividing people into compartments.

(McWhinney 1989)

Many models of health care have been described, reflecting historical developments and different philosophical viewpoints. An overview of these models provides an insight into the richness and diversity of medical practice and offers differing perspectives on human values, health, illness and disease, as well as on patients and doctors. Some of the main models are shown in Table 1. The models are not mutually exclusive, and there are considerable areas of overlap.

Table 1   **Models of health care**

- Biomedical (biomechanical) and biopsychosocial
- Reductionist and holistic (integrative)
- Disease-based and illness-based
- Patient-centred and population-centred
- Reactive and anticipatory
- Patient-centred and doctor-centred

Source: Stewart et al (1995)

Biomedical (biomechanical) and biopsychosocial

The biomedical or biomechanical model of health care has dominated medical practice in Western society. This traditional model, also known as the Oslerian model, after the famous early-20th century physician, Sir William Osler, sees the doctor as a scientist, applying expert knowledge and skills to medical problems. It is a model that focuses on disease, particularly physical or organic disease, the doctor acting like a medical detective to pinpoint the problem and then like a car mechanic to 'fix' it. Traditional medical education has been based on this model, which reinforces specialism, hospital-based medicine and a paternalistic view of medical practice.

In contrast, the biopsychosocial model acknowledges the importance of psychosocial, emotional and social factors alongside physical factors, recognising the interaction of all these factors in illness and disease (Engel 1980). This model extends the scientific basis of the biomedical model to encompass humanitarian aspects of the practice of medicine. The

---

Table 2   **Principles of professional practice**

Good clinical care

- Maintaining good medical practice
- Relationships with patients
- Working with colleagues
- Teaching and training
- Probity
- Health

Source: General Medical Council (2002)

---

biopsychosocial model is now replacing the biomedical model as the template for undergraduate medical education, as outlined in the General Medical Council's (2002) recommendations, 'Tomorrow's Doctors'. Table 2 summarises the principles of professional practice which must form the basis of medical education in the UK.

Reductionist and holistic (integrative)

The reductionist model of health care links with the traditional biomedical model. It reflects the 'scientific triumphalism' (Toon 1994) of the late Victorian period, suggesting that a systematic, objective and scientific approach can solve all problems. The model promotes the notion of separating out mind and body, designating problems as 'physical' or 'mental'. It encourages the traditional clinical method – detailed history-taking, physical examination and an investigation of each complaint (see pp 20–21). Excessive objectivity can, however, lead to treating patients as 'cases', and the reductionist approach risks missing the 'big picture' by focusing on fine details.

The holistic or integrative model encourages a broader, all-encompassing view of patients and their problems. This model promotes the notion of whole-person medicine, that is 'treating an illness as part of a problem in the whole of a person's life, rather than detaching it as a mechanical problem with the body to be fixed' (Toon 1994). It challenges the doctor-dominated biomedical and reductionist models by recognising that alternative practitioners and complementary therapies may have something to offer. Many patients and doctors are now acknowledging the benefits of acupuncture, homeopathy

and chiropractic as evidence of their effectiveness emerges.

Disease based (medical) and illness based (social)

The scientific basis of Western medical practice was established by the work of Laennec, Virchow and Pasteur. The disease-based model underpins the biomechanical and reductionist models. Since most of the significant advances in the doctor's ability to diagnose disease have come from linking the symptoms and signs of pathology, the disease-based model focuses on the physical. Although this is appropriate for many medical problems, it neglects the enormous contribution of cultural, social, spiritual and psychological factors to ill-health. The illness-based model acknowledges these factors and broadens the perspective of human suffering beyond that of simple organic dysfunction.

Patient centred and population centred

The patient-centred model focuses on the individual, highlighting the unique nature of the patient–doctor relationship. It is constructed around the consultation, described as 'the essential unit of medical practice' by Sir James Spence (1960). Although this model still lies at the core of personal clinical doctoring, it has to be considered alongside the bigger picture of the population-centred model.

Most of the major improvements in the health of nations have resulted from prevention and from better public health measures such as immunisation programmes, clean water, sanitation and improved housing. The population-centred model is favoured by public health doctors and aims to produce the greatest good for the greatest number of individuals. This is in direct conflict with the patient-centred approach and its emphasis on the individual and autonomy. A further issue that is becoming increasingly problematic as the cost of medical care increases is reconciling clinical freedom with finite health budgets. Clinicians in hospital and general practice consequently have to balance the patient-centred and population-centred approaches in their everyday practice.

Reactive and anticipatory

The traditional biomedical, disease-based, reductionist approach involves a reactive model in which the doctor responds to the symptoms or problems with which the patient has presented. The anticipatory model of health care recognises the importance of health promotion and aims to maximise the individual's health by primary, secondary and tertiary prevention (Table 3) (see also pp 30–35). As many issues concern life-style and behavioural change, the anticipatory model shifts responsibility for health back to the individual/patient and links with the biopsychosocial and holistic models.

Table 3	**The three levels of prevention**
First level	■ Immunisation
	■ Health education, e.g. advice on exercise, healthier eating or the use of condoms
Second level	■ Cervical screening
	■ Mammography
Third level	■ Stopping smoking in chronic obstructive airways disease
	■ Lipid-lowering drugs in coronary artery disease

Patient centred and doctor centred

Disciplines such as psychology, sociology and anthropology contribute to the patient-centred model of health care. This embraces the biopsychosocial and holistic models and encourages an adult-to-adult relationship between the patient and the doctor. In contrast, the traditional doctor-centred model is based on paternalism and perpetuates an adult–child relationship. The strong movement towards consumerism and the increased availability of medical and health-related information to the public (via books, magazine, television and the Internet) has challenged the doctor-centred model and many practitioners now view the consultation as a 'meeting between experts', the patient being acknowledged as an expert on

Table 4   The patient-centered clinical method

The six interactive components of the patient-centered process:

1. Exploring both the disease and the illness experience
   - ■ Differential diagnosis
   - ■ Dimensions of illness (ideas, feelings, expectations and effects on function)
2. Understanding the whole person
   - ■ The 'person' (life history and personal and developmental issues)
   - ■ The context (the family and anyone else involved in or affected by the patient's illness; the physical environment)
3. Finding common ground regarding management
   - ■ Problems and priorities
   - ■ Goals of treatment
   - ■ Roles of doctor and patient in management
4. Incorporating prevention and health promotion
   - ■ Health enhancement
   - ■ Risk reduction
   - ■ Early detection of disease
   - ■ Ameliorating effects of disease
5. Enhancing the patient–doctor relationship
   - ■ Characteristics of the therapeutic relationship
   - ■ Sharing power
   - ■ Caring and healing relationship
   - ■ Self-awareness
   - ■ Transference and countertransference
6. Being realistic
   - ■ Time
   - ■ Resources
   - ■ Team building

Source: Stewart et al (1995)

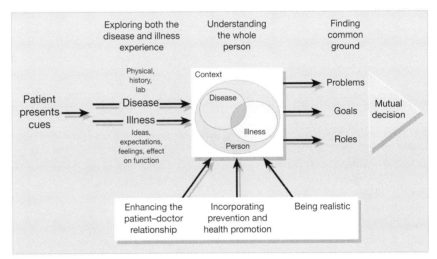

Fig. 1   **The patient-centred clinical method.** Source: Stewart et al (1995).

themselves, their background and feelings (Tuckett et al 1985).

Consequently, patient-centred medicine is becoming more established, and is forming a powerful alliance with evidence-based medicine (see pp 22–23), to the mutual benefit of both patient and doctors. Evidence-based, patient-centred medicine offers an opportunity to integrate the conventional understanding of disease with each patient's unique experience of illness (Stewart et al 1995), and addresses this through six interactive components (Table 4). The patient-centred clinical method is illustrated in Figure 1.

Models of health care

- ■ There is a huge diversity in models of health care.
- ■ These models reflect differing perspectives and viewpoints, and are not mutually exclusive, often overlapping.
- ■ Medical education is adapting to accommodate society's changing perspectives.
- ■ Evidenced-based, patient-centred medicine offers a model which accommodates multiple pespectives.

International comparisons I

Health-care systems are influenced by economic, cultural, religious, political, social and geographical factors. The interrelationships between the four levels of care and administration (see p. 2) and their associated funding systems determine many of the differences between countries. There are three main types of funding systems internationally (Fry and Horder 1994):

- *national health systems* – comprehensive and covering whole populations, financed and administered predominantly by governments
- *insurance-based schemes* – private or public, with varieties of service and coverage
- *multi-funded schemes* – including a mix of private insurance, personal expenditure and some government finance (either direct or reimbursement).

Despite these differences there are considerable similarities between countries in the clinical problems presenting in primary care and in common health indices (Table 1).

Morbidity studies have been conducted in a number of countries and demonstrate remarkable concurrence in the conditions presenting to primary care physicians. Table 2 shows the 10 most common presenting symptoms/conditions in six different countries. As mentioned on page 4 and 5, the content of primary care medicine is a mix of minor, self-limiting, chronic, non-curable and acute, major, life-threatening conditions. Despite these similarities, there are marked differences in the total health expenditure between different countries.

Expenditure

Figure 1 shows there is a nearly threefold difference between the highest (the USA) and the lowest (Luxembourg) spending countries. When expressed as total health expenditure per person, there is an almost fivefold difference between the highest and the lowest (Table 3).

There are a number of reasons for these large differences (Fry and Horder 1994):

- administrative expenses: 20% in the USA, 10% in Canada and 5% in the UK
- payments to physicians and other health staff (higher in the USA and Canada than in the UK)

Table 1 Demographics in 13 countries across Europe, North America and the Pacific Rim

Country	Population (%) Under 15	Population (%) Over 65	Crude birth rate (per 1000)	Total fertility rate per woman	Infant mortality rate per 1000 live births	Life expectancy years Male	Life expectancy years Female
USA	21.4	12.6	14.1	1.9	9.9	73	80
Sweden	17.3	18.1	12.6	1.9	5.7	75	81
Netherlands	18.3	12.7	12.9	1.6	7.1	74	81
Germany	16.0	14.9	10.9	1.5	7.5	73	79
Japan	18.4	11.7	11.5	1.7	6.0	76	82
Singapore	23.3	5.6	16.3	1.8	6.7	72	77
Hong Kong	20.7	8.8	12.3	1.4	6.9	75	80
Canada	20.9	11.4	12.9	1.7	7.3	74	81
Denmark	17.0	15.4	11.0	1.5	8.8	73	79
Spain	20.1	13.1	12.8	1.7	9.9	74	80
France	20.1	13.8	13.4	1.8	7.5	73	81
UK	19.0	15.4	13.7	1.8	7.4	73	79
Ireland	23.7	11.4	14.5	1.9	6.2	73	79

Source: Fry and Horder (1994)

Table 2 Most common presenting symptoms or conditions in primary care

England[1]	USA[2]	Canada[3] (males)	New Zealand[4]	Australia[5]	Japan[6]
Muscular aches	General medical examination	Cough	Prescription	Check-up	Influenza
Cough	Acute upper respiratory tract infection	Sore throat	Check-up	Prescription	Upper respiratory tract infection
Skin infection/irritation		Cold	Throat complaint	Cough	
Abdominal pain		Abdominal/pelvic pain	Pre-/postnatal check	Throat complaint	Gastritis
Diarrhoea/vomiting	Hypertension	Rash	Rash	Back complaint	Bronchitis
Sore throat/inflamed tonsils	Antenatal care	Fever/chill	Upper respiratory tract infection	Rash	Hypertension
Cold/blocked nose/sinus problems	Acute otitis media	Earache	Hypertension	Abdominal pain	Hyperlipidaemia
Back pain	Acute lower respiratory tract infection	Back problem	Back complaint	Immunisation	Diabetes mellitus
Breathlessness/wheezing	Acute sprains and strains	Skin inflammation	Headache	Headache	Hepatitis
Chest pain	Depression and anxiety	Chest pain	Abdominal pain	General weakness/tiredness	Lumbago
	Diabetes mellitus				
	Lacerations and contusions				

[1]Wilkin et al (1987), [2]Rosenblatt et al (1995), [3]Bass et al (1986), [4]McAvoy et al (1994), [5]Bridges–Webb et al (1992), [6]Kabayashi (1997)

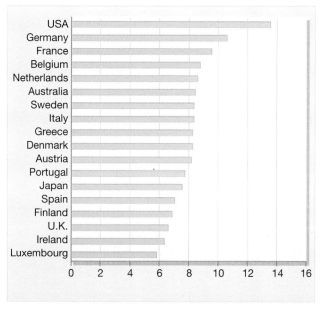

Fig. 1 **Total health expenditure (public and private) as a percentage of gross domestic product (GDP) 1998.** Source: Organisation for Economic Co-operation and Development (2001).

- use of high-technology services for diagnosis and treatment in the USA, Canada and UK
- medical and student manpower rates (Table 4)
- differences in demography (ageing populations) and the public demands and the expectations fostered by the media.

The cost of health care in developed nations is inversely proportional to the percentage of primary care physicians in the system. This is clearly seen by comparing the figures for the UK, Canada and the USA (Fig. 2). Within any country, developed or undeveloped, it has, however, repeatedly been demonstrated that no more than one-third of the variation in mortality rate can be attributed to the quality of medical care. Two-thirds of the variation is attributable to the distribution of income across a nation's population, the least well off dying much earlier than those better off.

World Health Report 2000

Building on Starfield's work (see p. 3) which showed the cost-effectiveness and patient acceptability of primary care orientated health-care systems, the World Health Organization has produced a report analysing the increasingly important influence of health systems in the daily lives of people world wide (WHO 2001).

Health systems in 191 member states were measured using five performance indicators:

- Overall level of population health
- Health inequalities (or disparities) within the population
- Overall level of health-system responsiveness (a combination of patient satisfaction and how well the system acts)
- Distribution of responsiveness within the population (how well people of varying economic status find that they are served by the health system)
- Distribution of the health system's financial burden within the population (who pays the cost).

Based on these performance indicators the best overall health care is provided by France, followed among major countries by Italy, Spain, Oman, Austria and Japan (Table 5). Although the USA spends the highest proportion of its gross domestic product on health in the world, its overall performance rates 37th amongst 191 countries. The

poorest performing countries are largely sub-Saharan African, where life expectations are low as a result of the AIDS epidemic.

Table 3 Total health expenditure per person in selected OECD countries 1998 (figures in American dollars)[1]

Country	$	Country	$
Portugal	859	Netherlands	1800
Greece	957	Canada	1828
Spain	1044	Ireland	1938
UK	1607	Sweden	2146
Australia	1696	Japan	2283
Belgium	1697	France	2358
Austria	1703	Denmark	2736
Italy	1720	Germany	2769
Finland	1724	USA	4178

Source: Organisation for Economic Co-operation and Development (2001)

[1]Includes private and public spending

Table 4 Active doctors per 1000 population, 1996

Country	Number per 1000 population	Country	Number per 10 000 population
UK	1.7	Luxembourg	3
Japan	1.9	France	3
Canada	2.1	Portugal	3.1
Ireland	2.2	Sweden	3.1[3]
Netherlands	2.6[1]	Belgium	3.4[2]
USA	2.7	Germany	3.5
Denmark	2.7[3]	Greece	4.1[4]
Austria	3	Spain	4.4
Finland	3	Italy	5.9

[1]1991, [2]1995, [3]1996, [4]1997

Source: Organisation for Economic Co-operation and Development (2001)

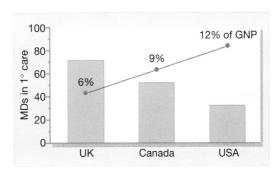

Fig. 2 **Inverse relationship between percent of primary care physicians and cost of health care as percent of Gross National Product (GNP).** Source: Rakel (1997)

Table 5 Sample of the WHO top 50 member nations in terms of overall health system performance

Rank	Country	Rank	Country
1	France	17	Netherlands
2	Italy	18	United Kingdom
3	San Marino	19	Ireland
4	Andorra	20	Switzerland
5	Malta		
6	Singapore		
7	Spain	41	New Zealand
8	Oman	42	Bahrain
9	Austria	43	Croatia
10	Japan	44	Qatar
11	Norway	45	Kuwait
12	Portugal	46	Barbados
13	Monaco	47	Thailand
14	Greece	48	Czech Republic
15	Ireland	49	Malaysia
16	Luxembourg	50	Poland

Source: WHO (2001)

International comparisons II

Workload

There is a considerable difference between countries in terms of consultation rate, length of consultation, hours worked and hospitalisation rates (Table 1). Consultations in Sweden last on average 2.5 times longer than those in the UK. German doctors work twice as many hours in direct patient care as do French doctors and see nearly three times as many patients. Moreover, the referral rate varies three-fold (Fig. 1) and the number of home visits in an average working week more than 40-fold across Europe (Fig. 2).

Services

Primary care physicians provide a range of services in different countries. Table 2 shows the percentage of services never or almost never provided by GPs in 15 European countries: a wide variation exists in the provision of all types of service. This is partly related to the degree of direct access the public has to specialist care, this ranging, as Table 3 shows, from none in UK to 82% in Germany.

The benefits of primary health care

As mentioned on page 3, Starfield (1992) has reviewed health care in 11 Western industrialized nations and concluded that a primary care orientation is associated with lower costs of care, higher satisfaction of the population with its health services, better health levels and lower medication use. The primary care orientation was characterized by a score derived from an average of scores on 11 different features of primary care – five being characteristics of the health system in general (Box 1) and six reflecting attempts of primary care practice to achieve a higher level of performance (Box 2). Figures 3 and 4 compare primary care scores and outcome indicators with primary care scores and health care expenditures in the 11 countries (Starfield 1994).

Table 1 **Primary care physicians' weekly consultations and hours, and hospitalisation rates**

Country	Consultations (face-to-face)	Consultation length	Hours worked in direct care (excluding on call) (estimated)	Annual hospitalisation (% population admissions)
USA	135	14.0[1] 18.0[2]	48	14
Sweden	100	20.0	42	18
Netherlands	150	7.5	45	11
Germany	220	–	55	22
Japan	325	–	57	14
Singapore	250	–	50	15(e)
Hong Kong	375	–	55	15(e)
Canada	140(e)	11–13.5	45	14
Denmark	100	–	32	21
Spain	150	–	30	9
France	82	13.7	25	22
Yugoslavia	–	5.0	–	–
Switzerland	–	12.5	–	–
UK	133	8.6	42	13

Source: Fry and Horder (1994)

[1]Family physicians, [2]Internists, (e) estimated

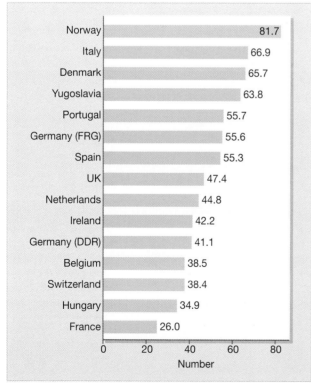

Fig. 1 **Referrals per 1000 consultations.** (Reproduced with the permission of the Royal College of General Practitioners. Source: RCGP 1992)

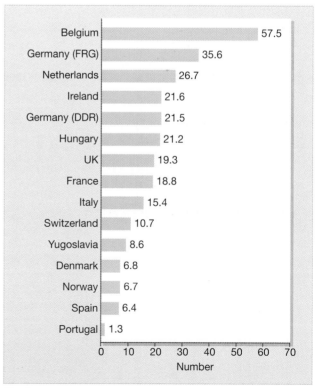

Fig. 2 **Number of home visits in an average working week.** (Reproduced with the permission of the Royal College of General Practitioners. Source: RCGP 1992)

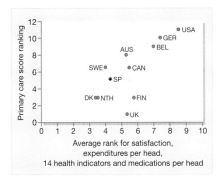

Fig. 3 **Primary care score versus 'outcome' indicators.** 1 = best; 12 = worst. Adapted from Starfield (1994).

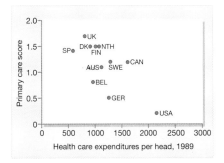

Fig. 4 **Primary care score versus health care expenditures.** Adapted from Starfield (1994).

Box 1 **Characteristics of the health system** (Starfield 1994)

- Universality of financial access to services
- Explicit regulation of distribution of health service resources to achieve or encourage equitable distribution
- Assignment of primary care function to one particular type of physician
- Earnings of primary care physicians relative to those of specialists
- Percentage of active physicians who are primary care physicians

---

Box 2 **Attempts of primary care practice to achieve a higher level of performance** (Starfield 1994)

- First contact care
- Longitudinality
- Comprehensiveness
- Coordination
- Family centredness
- Community orientation

Table 2 **Percentage of services never or almost never provided by 16 GPs in 15 European countries**

Country	Total (%)	Preventive and supportive (%)	Minor surgery (%)	X-ray (%)	Clinical laboratory (%)
Spain	80	41	100	90	93
Portugal	N/A	40	N/A	100	88
France	68	13	71	95	86
Italy	68	25	88	100	73
Austria	64	43	33	100	70
Republic of Ireland	59	8	14	100	76
Holland	55	12	50	100	60
Belgium	53	16	25	100	59
Great Britain	52	12	57	100	52
Sweden	45	7	13	100	33
Denmark (outside Copenhagen)	44	12	38	100	38
Denmark (Copenhagen)	41	9	25	100	33
Switzerland	33	0	29	55	44
Norway	25	0	17	80	10
West Germany	19	12	38	20	19
Finland	10	16	14	0	10
All countries	49	17	41	83	53

Source: Fry and Horder (1994)

Table 3 **Accessibility of health-care systems: the rate shows the proportion of specialist professions directly accessible to the public**

Rank order	Health-care system	Rate	Number (of relevant professions)
1	Federal Republic of Germany	0.82	33
2	Ireland S (medium/high income)	0.81	31
3	Belgium	0.79	33
4	Switzerland	0.78	32
	Finland S (private)	0.78	32
6	Sweden	0.74	34
7	Denmark, Copenhagen	0.68	34
8	France	0.65	34
9	Austria	0.62	31
10	Denmark outside Copenhagen	0.29	34
11	Portugal	0.18	32
12	Italy	0.15	33
13	The Netherlands (private)	0.13	34
16	Ireland (low income)	0.09	34
	The Netherlands (public)	0.09	34
	Norway	0.09	33
	Spain	0.09	33
18	Finland (public)	0.03	32
19	UK	0.00	32

Source: Fry and Horder (1994)

International comparisons

- Every country has its own individual health-care system
- There is considerable difference in funding systems, expenditure, workload and accessibility to services (both primary care and specialist) between countries
- There are remarkable similarities in the clinical problems or conditions presenting in primary care, and in basic health indices across countries
- There is a wide variation in overall performance of health-care systems, even among countries with similar levels of income and health expenditure
- In general, primary care-orientated health-care systems provide more cost-effective health care with greater patient satisfaction

Resources and needs: UK perspective I

Comparisons and differences between health-care systems around the world are outlined in pages 8–11; these sections focus on the resources and needs of the UK health system. The National Health Service (NHS) was established in 1948 and has undergone a series of major reforms during its lifetime. Over the past 50 years, general practice has passed through a number of 'ages' (Table 1), some more positive than others. Within the past 10 years, there has been a steady move towards a 'primary care-led NHS', offering considerable opportunities and responsibilities to GP.

Expenditure

In 1998–99, the total NHS expenditure was £39.8 billion, over 80% of this being raised from general taxation (Department of Health 2000). As mentioned on page 8, this represents 6.7% of gross domestic product (GDP), making the NHS very cost-effective compared with most other European countries and the USA (which spends 13.6% of its GDP). GP services account for less than 10% of this total, and prescribing for 13%, the majority being spent on hospital-based services.

The average cost of a general practice consultation is about £13, making the total cost for a patient's annual surgery visits approximately £63 in 1998/99 (Office of Health Economics 2000). The cost of prescribing is discussed on pages 86–87.

Workforce

The NHS workforce in England comprises 252 800 nurses, 349 300 managers and administrators, 56 100 hospital doctors and 31 000 GPs, the number of GPs having increased by 18% since 1985 (Department of Health 2000).

Most GPs are independent contractors, having a contract with their local health authority to provide 'general medical services' to a registered population. They are paid a gross income by the NHS, out of which they meet practice expenses, including such items as staff salaries, the cost of surgery premises and motoring expenses. The Doctors' and Dentists' Review Body is an independent body charged with advising the government on the appropriate level of pay for doctors and dentists working in the NHS. It

takes evidence from the professions and the Department of Health, making its recommendations directly to the Prime Minister. In 2001, average gross pay was £80 732 and average pay net of expenses was £56 610.

The payment system for GPs is a mix of capitation fees, fixed allowances and fees for a number of separate services. Practice expenses are partly included in these and partly reimbursed to individual GPs on the basis of the actual cost incurred. Capitation fees now account for 60% of NHS GPs' remuneration and are graded into three groups depending on the age of the patients.

There are a number of fixed allowances, the most important being the basic practice allowance (BPA). To qualify for this, a GP has to have at least 400 registered patients. The level of the BPA increases with the list size up to a ceiling of 1200 patients. The BPA is weighted in favour of lower list sizes and part-time GPs. Other allowances include a seniority allowance, dependent on the number of years in practice, a post-graduate education allowance, deprivation payments (related to the level of social deprivation in the practice) and allowances for teaching medical students and trainee GPs.

Fees for specified services include those for minor surgery, health promotion, child health surveillance, the examination of newly registered patients, contraceptive services, home visits at night (between 10 p.m. and 8 a.m.) and maternity services. There are also target payments for childhood immunisations and cervical cytology. A new contract is currently being negotiated which will be between a primary care organisation and a practice (rather than with an individual doctor), and services will be categorised as either essential, additional or enhanced (Lewis and

Gillam 2002). All GPs must provide essential services but will be able to reduce some of their current commitments.

The most recent rounds of health reforms have signalled a shift towards salaried employment and a range of more flexible working arrangements, including part-time work. This is consistent with recent changes in attitudes to life-style and work, and with an alteration in the demography of GPs. In 1999, 31.75% of GPs in England and Wales were women (compared with 17.4% in 1983), as were more than half of general practice registrars (Royal College of General Practitioners 2000). Approximately 40% of all female GPs, however, work part time, compared with about 6% of all male practitioners. In 1999, 67% of all GPs in England and Wales were aged 30–49, and almost 80% had been born in the UK. One in four GPs has a part-time hospital appointment as a clinical assistant.

Organisation of general practice

There are about 11 000 practices in the UK, most GPs working in partnerships. In 1997, only 10% of GPs were single handed, 28.5% working in practices of six or more doctors. Thirteen and a half per cent of GPs are dispensing doctors, providing medicines and appliances to patients living more than 1 mile from a pharmacy.

GPs provide a single entry point into the NHS (apart from accident and emergency cases, sexually transmitted diseases and some family planning and occupational health services). They provide 24 hour access and availability, as well as first contact care involving diagnosis, assessment, triage and the management or resolution of all defined problems. This involves co-ordinating local medical and social

Table 1 **The ages of NHS general practice**	
The Dark Ages 1948–1966	■ Single handed and on call at all times
	■ Home as surgery and wife as receptionist
	■ Income from capitation only
The Renaissance 1966–1986	■ Group practices and primary health-care teams
	■ Better premises
	■ Academic departments
The Reformation 1986–1990	■ New GP contract
	■ NHS reforms
Modern Times 1990–	■ Strategic shift to primary care

Source: Harrison and van Zwanenberg (1998)

services and operating a gatekeeping function through selective referrals. GPs also have responsibility for disease prevention, health maintenance and promotion, immunisation, screening for cervical cytology and breast cancer, and check-ups of new patients and all those aged 75 years and over.

Most GPs employ practice nurses, secretaries, receptionists and practice managers; they work closely with community nurses, health visitors and midwives. Together, these form the primary health-care team. Over the years, the professional mix of such teams has tended to expand, and this trend is likely to continue (Fig. 1). The number of staff working in general practice has risen by a fifth over the past 5 years (Royal College of General Practitioners 1999). Between 1984 and 1994, there was a significant growth in the number of nurses in primary care. Over that period, the number of practice nurses rose from around 1900 to just over 9000, that of community psychiatric nurses from 1800 to nearly 4800 and the number of nurses specialising in the care of people with learning disabilities from 770 to over 2000 (Secretary of State for Health 1996). Primary health-care services are also provided by pharmacists, optometrists, dentists and therapy services (physiotherapists, occupational therapists, speech and language therapists, and chiropodists).

The structure and organisation of general practice and primary care services have been radically altered in the latest health reforms, primary care groups (PCGs) being seen as the vehicle for driving through a major shift in emphasis from secondary and tertiary care to primary care. The practice-based primary health care team (PHCT) is seen as the basic unit of care in the community. The functions of the PHCT as defined by the RCGP are shown in Table 2.

General practitioners with special interests

A recent innovation identified in the NHS Plan (see p. 15) is the development of up to 1000 'specialist GPs' to take referrals from their colleagues for a range of conditions. These general practitioners with special interests (GPwSIs) are intended to provide additional opportunities for GPs to work in new ways that will enhance their skills and improve career opportunities. This initiative is also intended to improve management

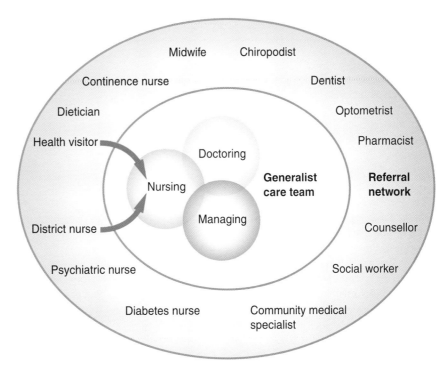

Fig. 1 **Model of the future primary care team and the surrounding specialist network of services in the community.** Source: Royal College of General Practitioners (1996).

Table 2 **Functions of the Primary Health Care Team**

- The diagnosis and management of acute and chronic conditions, treatment in emergencies, when necessary in the patient's home
- Antenatal and postnatal care, and access to contraceptive advice and provision
- Prevention of disease and disability
- The follow-up and continuing care of chronic and recurring disease
- Rehabilitation after illness
- Care during terminal illness
- The coordination of services for those at risk, including children, the mentally ill, the bereaved, the elderly, the handicapped and those who care for them
- Helping patients and their relatives to make appropriate use of other agencies for care and support including hospital-based specialists

Source: Royal College of General Practitioners (1992)

of workload between primary and secondary care and enhance the quality of referrals to consultants (Department of Health/Royal College of General Practitioners 2002).

GPwSIs are meant to supplement their important generalist role by delivering a high quality, improved access service to meet the needs of a single Primary Care Trust or group of PCTs. They may deliver a clinical service beyond the normal scope of general practice, undertake advanced procedures or develop services. However, they do not offer a full consultant service and will not replace consultants or interfere with access to consultants by local GPs. Their roles will be circumscribed but within their role definition they should offer a high quality service. The areas considered most likely to be priorities in terms of national programs or services with significant access problems are shown in Box 1.

Box 1 **Priority areas for GPs with special interests (DOH/RCGP 2002)**

- Cardiology
- Care of the elderly
- Diabetes
- Palliative care and cancer
- Mental health (including substance misuse)
- Dermatology
- Musculoskeletal medicine
- Women and child health, including sexual health
- Ear, nose and throat
- Care for the homeless, asylum seekers, travellers and others who find access to traditional health services difficult
- Other procedures suitable for community settings (endoscopy, echocardiography, vasectomy, etc.)

Resources and needs: UK perspective II

Workload

The average list size of a GP in 2000 was 1787 patients, 10% less than in 1986. In total, UK GPs conduct about 269 million consultations each year, an increase of almost 50% since 1975 and 15.9% since 1985 (Royal College of General Practitioners 2001). Eighty per cent of the population consult their GP at least once per year, this rising to 90% over a 5 year period. Of those attending, each patient visits his or her GP on average four times per year. This is equivalent to about 740 000 people (approximately 1.3% of the population) consulting a GP every day. Women tend to consult GPs more often than men.

GPs spend an average of just over 39 hours per week on general medical duties, rising to 58 hours when on-call work is included. They will conduct on average 154 consultations per week, 84% of these in the surgery. The average surgery consultation lasts 9.36 minutes, home visit (including travelling time) taking 25.2 minutes on average. Sixty-nine per cent of consultations involve issuing a prescription, and 13% of cases are referred to secondary care.

Training and education

Mandatory vocational training for general practice was introduced in 1982. This involves 3 years' approved post-graduate experience, usually 2 years in hospital posts such as paediatrics, obstetrics, psychiatry and general medicine and 1 year in 'apprenticeship' in general practice as a 'registrar' or 'trainee'.

Once established in practice, doctors are expected to maintain their knowledge and skills by continuing medical education or professional development, financial rewards being provided for those GPs undertaking approved educational activities. The current system is fragmented, is largely uniprofessional and does not address true educational needs. A recent review has recommended practice professional development plans, which would integrate and improve the educational process and encourage multi-disciplinary learning within the practice team. In addition, a system of periodic revalidation for all medical practitioners is due to be introduced by the General Medical Council in the near future.

The changing nature of general practice – the new NHS

A number of strategic themes developed within the NHS during the 1990s (Table 1), a major one being greater influence for GPs. These themes reflected demographic and political changes such as an ageing population, a shift towards more chronic disease, a re-direction of health-care emphasis from the hospital to the community, an encouragement of the public to expect more from the health services and pressure to de-regulate professional monopolies (Harrison and van Zwanenberg 1998).

The strategic shift to primary care began in the early 1990s, empowering GPs by means of fund-holding, locality commissioning and total purchasing. These different methods of controlling budgets and purchasing secondary care services gave GPs a much greater say in the organisation and delivery of their local health services, but participation in them was voluntary. The NHS plans vary somewhat between the countries of the UK and here we deal primarily with the plans for England. The most recent reforms have established PCGs, which, unlike previous options, are mandatory and universal, with a uniform structure and progressive responsibilities (Baker 1998). The key features of PCGs are shown in Table 2. By 2004 all PCGs are expected to have achieved the top (4th) level of responsibility and to have become Primary Care Trusts.

A number of other features of these reforms have major implications for general practice:

- *National targets.* These are described in the 1998 policy paper on public health, 'Our Healthier Nation' (Department of Health 1998). They focus on five major causes of mortality and morbidity (heart disease, stroke, accidents, cancer and mental health) and form the basis of health improvement programmes.
- *Health improvement programmes.* These are action programmes to improve health and health care locally and are led by the health authority, which will involve NHS Trusts, PCGs and other primary care professionals working in partnership with the local authority and engaging other local interests. The programmes will be 3 year rolling plans with annual updates.
- *National Institute for Clinical Excellence.* This was established as a special health authority in April 1999 with three broad functions:
  - the appraisal of new and existing health technologies
  - the development of clinical guidelines
  - the promotion of clinical audit and confidential enquiries.
- *Health action zones.* These involve bringing together organisations within and beyond the NHS to develop and implement a locally agreed strategy for improving the health of local people, especially in areas of deprivation and health inequality. Eleven health action zones were established in April 1998 and a further 15 in April 1999, focusing on public health and community care initiatives.
- *Clinical governance.* This is a system through which NHS organisations are accountable for continuously improving the quality of their services and safeguarding high standards of care by creating an environment in which excellence in clinical care will flourish. This is an ambitious concept, embracing culture, infrastructure, coherence, quality methods, risk avoidance

---

Table 1 **Strategic themes in the NHS in the 1990s**

- Value for money
- Quality
- Engaging with patients
- More influence for GPs
- More community-based services

Table 2 **Key features of primary care groups**

- Responsibility for developing primary and community health care
- GPs and nurses in lead role, with support from pharmacists, managers and patients
- Cover approximately 100 000 population (50 GPs)
- Increasing range of responsibilities (four levels) – working with health authorities
- Ambitious agenda and timetable

Source: Harrison and van Zwanenberg (1998)

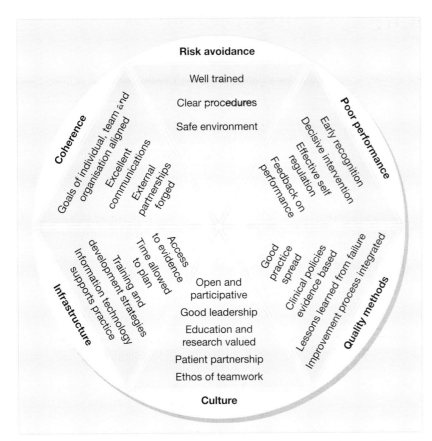

Fig. 1 **Integrating approaches from clinical governance.** (Adapted from Scally and Donaldson 1998.)

Table 4 **The NHS Plan's 10 priorities for improving health and social care**
- Cancer
- Coronary heart disease
- Mental health
- Children
- Older people
- Public health and reducing inequality
- Faster and easier access to services
- Workforce
- Quality
- IT, equipment and buildings

Source: Secretary of State for Health (2001)

and poor performance (see p. 17). Figure 1 illustrates the integrating approach of clinical governance.

On the 50th anniversary of the NHS in 1998, the Secretary of State, the NHS Executive and the royal colleges agreed on a new set of eight principles of progress for the NHS – the Langlands Eight (Table 3).

The NHS Plan

This is a 10-year strategy for bringing the NHS up to the standards that patients and staff want and expect in a 21st century health service. There are three main groups who are leading the changes, which were published in 2001:

- The Modernisation Board– comprising senior health and social care professionals and patient representatives
- The Modernisation Agency– supporting staff and managers in

the NHS to modernise services, helping underperforming organisations and developing the current and future leaders and managers of the health service
- Taskforces–involving front line professionals and patient representatives, spearheading progress across the NHS Plan's priority areas (Table 4).

General practice co-ops

The establishment of general practice co-operatives (co-ops) is a response by GPs to the burgeoning demands of out-of-hours care and is an attempt to make it manageable and bearable. GPs in large towns and cities could rely on deputising but many would still work 30–40 hours on call, especially in rural areas. The establishment and resourcing of out-of-hours co-ops has meant that in the UK a patient may ring NHS Direct for advice and, if necessary, be routed through to the doctor. Stress levels, which were dangerously high among GPs, have fallen with the advent of co-ops. Time spent on-call has been reduced and its awaiting improved. Students should try and gain experience in an out of hours co-op during their practice attachments.

Table 3 **The eight principles for progress for the NHS**

- Improvement comes from knowledge
- Measurement for improvement is not measurement for judgment
- Make control over care as local as possible
- Improvement requires cooperation among disciplines
- Waste is poor quality; removing waste is improvement
- Waiting costs more than it saves
- Service is at the care of our work
- Patients and families can care for themselves

Source: Berwick (1998)

Resources and needs: UK perspective
- GPs occupy the front line of clinical care.
- Ninety per cent of episodes of illness presenting to GPs are managed entirely within primary care.
- GP services account for less than 10% of total NHS expenditure.
- Ninety per cent of GPs work in groups.
- A minimum of 3 years approved post-graduate training is required before entering general practice.
- The 1990s has seen a strategic shift to primary care, GPs taking on greater responsibilities for the planning and delivery of care.

Professional standards

The duties of a doctor

The usual relationship between a doctor and a patient has some similarity to ordinary daily social interactions, but it also has some very distinctive features that make it a professional rather than a purely social relationship. All relationships with experts (for example, lawyers or financial advisers) are to an extent one sided because knowledge confers power. In the case of the doctor, that power can frequently be over life or death. Patients have to trust that their doctors are at least as good as other doctors in terms of knowledge and skill and that they are not acting beyond the limits of their competence.

During the 'privileged intimacy' of the consultation, many social norms are temporarily suspended while the patient discloses to the doctor information that he or she might not give even to their dearest companion, and may tacitly co-operate in physical contact of a kind that is generally limited to sexual partners. What might otherwise be a bizarre encounter usually proceeds smoothly because both sides recognise it to be an extraordinary relationship: a professional (as opposed to social) relationship, governed by ethical imperatives and constraints, whose function is to benefit the patient. Arising from this special relationship, the patient must also be able to trust that the doctor will not abuse it by, for example, giving away confidences, obtaining money or sexual favours, or deceiving the patient by making false claims about treatments or particularly by advertising these (like the old American wild west 'snake doctors').

Self-regulation has classically been taken to be a central tenet of the definition of a profession. Each doctor is expected to adhere to a code of professional ethics, the earliest example being the Hippocratic oath much of which still applies even though it dates from the time of Ancient Greece.

Professional regulation in the UK

In Britain, the British Medical Association (BMA) promoted the Medical Act of 1868, with the purpose 'that persons requiring medical aid should be able to distinguish qualified from unqualified practitioners'

(British Medical Association 1993), and the General Medical Council (GMC) was established to maintain a register of qualified practitioners and lay down minimum standards of medical education. The GMC possesses the power to suspend or remove doctors from the register for serious breaches of the professional code of ethics.

Main ethical principles

The main generally accepted ethical principles governing the professional relationship between doctor and patient have been described as follows:

- *Non-maleficence/beneficence* – the twin duties not only to do no harm to patients, but also, where possible, positively to do good towards them (and mankind in general).
- *Respect for autonomy* – the duty to respect each individual's right to choose and act as he or she wishes within the framework of the law and other proper constraints (which may include not offending the rights of other individuals).
- *Justice* – the duty to be as fair as possible to all individuals concerned, both in the distribution of resources (e.g. by seeing that your expertise is justly distributed between all the patients under your care) and in respecting the demands of individual rights.

These principles may conflict and often require to be integrated to form a balanced judgement. Justice, for example, requires that the demands of beneficence and autonomy in the case of one individual may need to be balanced against the requirements of others. In major accidents, for example, when medical expertise may initially be in short supply, a single-handed doctor might have to concentrate on saving the lives of those who are most likely to survive at the expense of the obviously dying.

To respect a person as an autonomous being is to take into account in your own conduct that you are dealing with another independent person. In effect, the duties of *non-maleficence/ beneficence* and of *justice* follow on

---

from the supreme principle of *respect for persons*. Put in another way, if your predominant *attitude* is always to respect autonomy, the other principles will tend to show almost automatically in the actions that you take.

The principle of autonomy of individuals is the cornerstone of a free society. In essence, it means treating people as free agents with the same right to choices and actions as we ourselves would wish to have in a free society. It means accepting people for what they are and respecting that they may have different attitudes and beliefs, and that they may choose to live in ways that we might not ourselves choose. It means not making value judgements about these differences and not acting towards others in a way that is judgemental. Nonetheless, there are situations in which an individual is not autonomous (for example, with children and the severely mentally handicapped), so others may have to make decisions for them. There are also limitations to autonomy, mainly the acceptability of the effects of individual actions on other people: these limitations are applied primarily through social pressure and the law of the land.

The main features of a good professional relationship are mutual feelings of respect and trust, which are in turn largely based on the quality of *empathy*, that is the ability to understand the predicament of others (and respect their personal autonomy), without necessarily *sympathising*, that is, feeling sorry for them. Our own moral and political beliefs should not intrude into the doctor–patient relationship. We are there to help, not to approve or disapprove. Particular examples of when such a dispassionate view is essential include dealing with drug and alcohol addiction, the issues surrounding abortion, marital infidelity and behavioural problems in children, especially where these seem to be associated with poor parenting.

Most universities now have ethical codes for medical students which reflect these principles (Box 3).

Clinical governance

Clinical governance (Royal College of General Practitioners 1999) is the latest concept in the development of professional control and regulation. It is essentially a framework, promoted by the National Health Service (NHS) (Department of Health 2000), for the improvement of patient care through a

professional commitment to high standards, reflective practice, risk management and personal and team development. Most of these concepts are well established, but clinical governance strengthens them and brings them together in an integrated structure.

Without going into detail, each tier of the structure of the NHS will be responsible for promoting clinical governance so that, in general practice for example, it will be the responsibility of each practice and, leading on from that, each group of practices, for example primary care groups (PCGs) in England and local health-care co-operatives in Scotland. It is envisaged that these bodies will collect information about the work of individual doctors (e.g. on prescribing

habits, referrals to hospital, etc) in order to monitor standards of care and intervene when it is though that a doctor may be 'underperforming' in comparison with the general standard of others. It is easy to see how most of these concepts derive from the fundamental principles of non-maleficence/beneficence, respect for autonomy and justice.

The overall concept is in fact very similar to the industrial framework of total quality management. It is the philosophy that the quality of work can always be improved, that we must continually learn in order to improve, and that mistakes must be carefully examined to avoid them in the future, in an atmosphere of the acceptance of human and systems failure rather than of blame.

Box 3 Duties of a medical student

Medical students have privileged access to patients and to information on patients. Each student has an obligation to be mentally and physically healthy enough to work with patients and to become a member of medical profession.

The student has a duty:
- To listen to patients, respect their views, treat patients politely and considerately, respect confidentiality and recognise the right of patients to refuse to take part in teaching
- Not to allow personal views about a patient's lifestyle, culture, beliefs, race, colour, gender, sexuality, age, social status, or perceived economic worth to prejudice interactions with patients, teachers or colleagues
- Not to abuse patients trust by, for example, forming improper personal relationships with patients or close relative
- Not to misrepresent him/herself as a qualified doctor.
- To maintain appropriate standards of dress, appearance and personal hygiene
- To physically examine patients in order to establish a clinical diagnosis
- To write legibly so that information can be communicated to colleagues
- To be able to undertake basic and advanced life support during the house officer year
- To ensure that vision is adequate to understand written instructions, names and dosages of drugs
- Of confidentiality to patients' records, data, and information about teachers and fellow students

Source: Based on criteria laid down by Birmingham University, UK, which also includes absence of dyslexia, adequate hearing and being fit-free in the preceding 12 months

---

Professional standards

- The relationship between doctor and patient is different from ordinary social relationships
- In a professional relationship the professional is in a position of power because of his or her special expertise. Therefore, there must be strict codes of conduct to protect patients against abuse of this power
- The main ethical principles are of non-maleficence/beneficence, respect for autonomy and justice
- Empathy, the development of mutual respect and trust, and holding all information in complete confidence are main examples of how these principles operate in practice
- Clinical governance is a recent development of these concepts, in which there is an integrated structure within the NHS that will help deliver high professional standards

Understanding the consultation

Although some consultations in general practice are quite simple for a student observer to understand, many are highly complex and bewildering for the newcomer. This section is intended to give you an elementary understanding of the main underlying processes.

The consultation

On average, a GP conducts about 40 consultations per day in his or her surgery and in addition visits about five people at home. As well as this 'face-to-face' time, there is a great deal of organisational and administrative work involved in running the practice and arranging further care for individual patients, which we will not consider here. The 5–7 minutes which was traditionally allocated for each consultation is proving increasingly inadequate, and many GPs are moving to 10 minute appointments to allow for the increased complexity of modern medicine. Within this framework, time is used flexibly so that simple problems are dealt with in a shorter time, allowing a greater amount of time to be spent with individuals who need it.

The duration of individual consultations ranges from 2 to 20 minutes. A consultation is often simply one of a series of contacts about the same episode of illness (the 'extended consultation') and one of a much larger series of contacts with the same patient. In the UK at least (as opposed to, for example, USA), the GP tends to deal with more complex problems in a series of small 'bites' over time rather than attempting to resolve the problem immediately, although the total amount of time spent with the patient for a particular episode of illness may be about the same. The difference between the UK and USA in this respect is partly the result of differences in methods of payment. The UK method, however, allows the evolution or resolution of symptoms over time to be taken into account, thereby avoiding initial intensive investigations, whereas the American system is bound to depend upon intensive 'on-the-spot' investigation and increased expense, a certain amount of which may be avoidable.

Figure 1 gives a simple classification of the kinds of problem dealt with, but

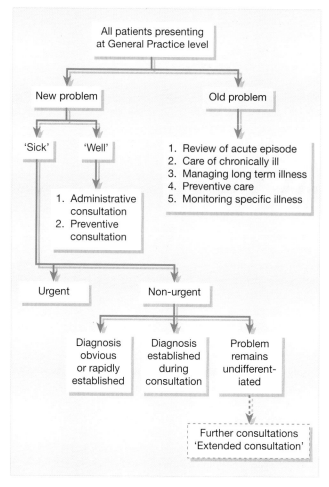

Fig. 1 **Types of problem dealt with.**

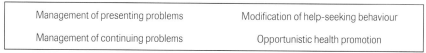

| Management of presenting problems | Modification of help-seeking behaviour |
| Management of continuing problems | Opportunistic health promotion |

Fig. 2 **The potential in each primary care consultation.** Source: Stott and Davis (1979).

it is quite usual for the patient to present several problems (both 'new' and 'old') to be dealt with at the same consultation. Stott and Davis (1979) identified four broad tasks (Fig. 2), some or all of which the doctor is attempting to carry out in each consultation.

Communication

High-quality medical practice depends not just on clinical knowledge and the conventional skills of history-taking and clinical examination: good clinicians are distinguished by their high level of interpersonal skills. Some patients rarely, if ever, consult a doctor, but a GP will in time come to be acquainted with most of his patients – some of course more than others. The quality of the relationship that the

doctor is able to build up over time is of considerable diagnostic and therapeutic importance. Patients are more likely to confide in someone whom they know and trust, so that they will be less likely to omit important information for reasons of delicacy or confidentiality. There is also evidence that compliance with recommended therapy is much improved by a good doctor–patient relationship and that the relationship itself is frequently an important part of the treatment.

It is unlikely that a good relationship can be built up where the quality of communication is poor. Indeed, it has been convincingly shown that the quality of the information that the doctor obtains from the patient relates very closely to the doctor's communication style. The doctor who listens attentively and empathetically will, for example, more frequently identify underlying psychological and/or social problems and avoid pursuing the blind alley of a misleading physical presenting symptom, such as recurrent headaches. Conversely, it may be necessary to control the flow of irrelevant information from the patient: one way of doing this is by being deliberately inattentive. The main point is that if you are aware of the various components of communication, and of how they can be used to good effect, it is certainly possible to enhance whatever natural ability you have by training and practice.

Clinical method is based on *observation* as well as communication, and the best clinicians in all fields of medicine are always highly observant people. They notice things that other clinicians miss, often because they are more alert to visual cues, incongruities in the patient's story or manner of telling it, and other unconventional sources of information such as the patient's environment – the state of his or her home or bedside locker, what he or she is reading, a full ashtray and so on. Various studies have shown that, even in hospital practice, about two-thirds of cases could in retrospect have been accurately diagnosed on the basis of history and simple observation or examination alone: 'Listen to the patient – he will tell you the diagnosis'.

Understanding human behaviour

Good clinicians also understand human behaviour. Social scientists study human behaviour in a scientific way and we cannot pretend to have their depth of knowledge but, particularly in general practice, knowing 'what makes people tick' is as fundamental as knowledge of anatomy or physiology.

One problem is that, whilst we may have no experience of anatomy and physiology, and therefore recognise that we must study these subjects, we all of us have experience of dealing with other people and may feel that further study is superfluous. We have developed intuitive ways of dealing with people which may seem successful enough. We may even think that we are 'good with people'. However, it is important to underpin good intuitive understanding with scientific knowledge from the social

sciences. It is particularly important to avoid *prejudice and 'jumping to conclusions'*, keeping an open mind. This shows itself in different ways. A commonly quoted example of pre-judgement is where a roughly dressed tramp found collapsed on the street is usually assumed to be drunk. If he were well dressed the first assumption would be more likely to be that he had had a stroke or a heart attack. Neither prior assumption is necessarily justified but it can colour our subsequent actions. These presumptions can affect the process of a consultation, e.g. a person who speaks ungrammatically or expresses themselves poorly might wrongly be assumed to be unintelligent. Another effect is to generate negative feelings towards the person, e.g. people who have difficulty altering risk-taking behaviour like drug-taking, smoking and being overweight may be regarded as stupid or in some way defective. These feelings may be particularly generated by drug addicts and alcoholics. It is especially important to overcome prejudicial attitudes that may interfere with our fair dealing with patients, i.e. not to stereotype

individuals unfavourably, even although that stereotyping may occasionally prove correct!

Any detailed discussion of social science is outwith the scope of this book (see our sister publication *Psychology and Sociology Applied to Medicine*, 1999 (Porter et al.) but other concepts that are important to communication within the consultation include *cognitive dissonance* (Box 1) and *attribution errors* (Box 2).

Box 1   Cognitive dissonance

This concept tries to help us understand why behaviour and attitudes can be totally at odds with one another in the same individual. For example a very heavy drinker/smoker or drug taker may well understand and believe that their behaviour is damaging to their health, but they continue the habit. Theories of cognitive dissonance are important in health promotion and education (see pp 30–35).

Box 2   Attribution errors

Attribution refers to the way that we try to understand the underlying motives for individual behaviour. For example, if we fail a job interview or examination, we might wonder what the reasons were – were they internal, to do with us, or external, to do with the employer or the examiners, for example? However, a number of well established biases affect attribution, for example:

The *fundamental attribution error* is that we naturally have a tendency to explain the actions of others in terms of disposition (internal) rather than situational (external) factors. Even although we know that situational forces like poverty and broken relationships adversely affect health, we may still sneakily feel that people have 'brought it on themselves'.

The *actor–observer effect* – 'You tripped; I was pushed'. We assume that our own behaviour arises from external causes but that of others is internal, e.g. their own clumsiness.

The *self-serving bias* – 'We, unlike others, can do no wrong'. We tend to credit success to internal factors and failure to external factors.

Understanding the consultation

- GPs see around 40–50 patients per day each in an average time of 7 minutes although individual times range to 20 minutes or more.
- Also, complex problems are commonly dealt with in an 'extended consultation' — a series of encounters over time

Clinical method in general practice: an overview

An introduction to clinical problem-solving

Between the steps of gathering information about the patient and giving advice and/or treatment, there lies an intermediate problem-solving process. Even though you are just starting your medical education, a simple introduction to this process is important because, even though much use is made of the specialised knowledge that you will gain in later years, the intellectual processes you will employ are not very different from those which most people use to solve everyday problems.

We will first try to illustrate the processes commonly involved by using non-medical analogies, but please bear in mind that such analogies can only ever be crude even though they should help you to understand the overall concept.

Pattern recognition

Suppose you park your car in a crowded multi-storey car park. When you get back, you find that the front bumper and an associated light cluster has been damaged. From the pattern of damage and the circumstances, it *looks* as if another car has damaged yours while trying to park, and this will be your most likely conclusion (even though there are other improbable possibilities). This is problem-solving at its simplest – you recognise a pattern that almost always implies a particular cause. Doctors use pattern recognition in a similar way, particularly in diagnosing common disorders of the skin. Childhood eczema, for example, has a distinctive appearance and distribution, affecting mainly the flexures of the wrists, the elbows and the backs of the knees.

Hypothetico-deductive reasoning

Next, suppose that you get into your car one cold winter's morning, turn the key and it makes a perfunctory noise and fails to start. There are many possible reasons why a car won't start, but some are more common, and therefore more *probable*, than others. The most probable reasons are (a) that you've run out of petrol and (b) that the battery is flat. To start with, (b) is already more likely than (a): even if there were no petrol at all, the battery would still make the engine turn and attempt to start. If you still aren't sufficiently convinced that a flat battery

is the cause, there are a few pieces of vital information that will clinch your 'diagnosis'. If, on the one hand, the headlights are very dim, this makes it much more likely that the battery is at fault; if, on the other, you can establish that there is petrol in the tank you have eliminated the main alternative cause. If you now attach jump leads to the car and it starts, this 'response to treatment' is further confirmation that the battery is faulty.

This is very like the hypothetico-deductive model that doctors intuitively use to solve a variety of common problems (Fig. 4). Intermittent brief chest pains, for example, may result from a variety of causes, arising from the muscles or skeleton, from the gullet (usually because of a reflux of acid from the stomach) or of course from the heart. Pain arising from the heart usually gets worse on exercise. Musculoskeletal pain will tend to be associated with tenderness of the affected muscles or joints, or will be worse on movements that stretch these structures, and pain arising from acid reflux in the gullet will tend to be associated with other features and a history of indigestion. These (and many other) associated findings help the doctor to identify the most likely cause, progressively confirm it and eliminate the other possible causes.

The response to treatment may also help the diagnosis. Transient heart pains (angina) will, for example, respond to glyceryl trinitrate, and although acid reflux in the gullet may also appear to respond to this, it usually responds much better to anti-acid treatments.

There are some important points to note here. First, the conclusion you reached is very likely to be correct, but there is a small possibility that it could be wrong. There are a large number of unusual causes of electrical faults in cars: to be absolutely sure, you would have to go to a great deal of time and expense to get an exhaustive check of the complete electrical system. Is this worth it? Why not wait and see what happens next? If there is an uncommon fault, it will almost certainly start to cause new and/or recurrent problems, and you have lost nothing by waiting.

Second, you hardly looked at the battery even though you decided that this was the source of the problem.

You could have measured its remaining electrical charge. Although an objective measurement like this would have established the cause very firmly, most of us do not have the necessary equipment, and it is sufficiently accurate, and definitely cheaper, to deduce the cause from indirect information, as you did here. In medicine, it is often the case, not just that expensive equipment is needed to obtain direct measurements, but that there is no satisfactory way of obtaining these anyway.

Third, once you decided that the battery was the most likely cause, you assumed that there was no other additional problem. Could there be more than one cause? There could be, but the chance of more than one fault arising simultaneously is very remote, and there was no evidence here to indicate a second cause. In the first instance at least, the best course is to assume a single cause.

The important points about hypothetico-deductive reasoning are therefore as follows:

- *Some causes are more probable than others*. Although it is efficient to bear the common causes uppermost in our minds, we also have to hold at the back of our minds the important, albeit rare, alternatives. Some of these may have to be positively excluded even although they are unlikely (usually because they might have immediately serious effects, meningitis being a good example).
- *Some pieces of information are more valuable than others*. A very few pieces of information are in fact often crucial, whereas other information may add relatively little to solving the problem.

Inductive reasoning

In the last example, you had from the beginning a good idea of what might be wrong. But suppose that you had *no idea* at all. For example, while you are driving happily along, the car suddenly starts to pour out black smoke, make loud and irregular noises and run very unevenly, before stopping completely. A car fanatic might possibly have an idea of what is wrong, but most of us wouldn't have the faintest notion. So how do we set about solving this sort of problem? First, since we have no idea what might be wrong, we don't know what

Table 1 **Clinical problem-solving – points to watch**

Stage	Points to watch
Presenting symptoms	Awareness of cues
	Premature 'closing off'
Initial hypothesis	Adequacy of hypothesis generation
	Awareness of differential probability
	Awareness of the most important *rare* possibilities to be excluded
	Ability to generate social and psychological as well as physical hypotheses
Data-gathering	Alertness to unconventional as well as conventional cues
	Accuracy of clarification
	Ability to discriminate
Hypothesis-testing	Ability to relate data to a knowledge of disease patterns
	Ability to assess weight of evidence
Revise initial hypotheses	Willingness to 'change track' and retrace steps if necessary
Provisional (working) diagnosis	Ability to assess the point at which a *safe* working diagnosis has been reached
	Ability to assess how much investigation is appropriate in the patient's best interests

This framework is primarily intended for use in discussion with tutors after, for example, observing a typical consultation

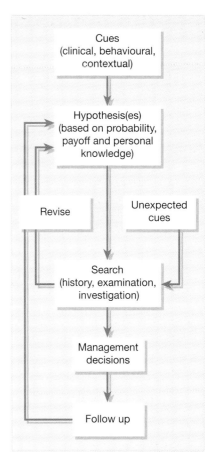

Fig. 1 **Model of the diagnostic process.**
Source: Barber (1975)

the most important pieces of evidence or information might be; indeed, we don't even know where to start. The only thing we can do is to adopt a *systematic* and *comprehensive* approach in which we (or more probably in this circumstance a mechanic) examine every mechanical system of the car in turn, looking for possible faults.

The ubiquitous complaint of constant tiredness ('tired all the time') is a good example of a situation in which this approach is required. There are so many possible causes – from physical causes such as chronic infection or diseases of the blood, to psychological ones, like depressive illness – that it may be difficult to find a starting point.

This is very like the way in which you will learn clinical method later in the medical course. It takes quite a lot of experience to be able to use the hypothetico-deductive model safely and effectively. To begin with, you will, in almost all cases, have no idea of what might be wrong, and you must therefore use the comprehensive inductive model. It is also the best way of learning about clinical method because it gives you a great deal of practice in all the various skills that are involved.

Caveats

This is of course a deliberate simplification, any similarity between cars and human beings being in reality very superficial. For a start, there is much more variation in the 'specification' of human beings. The size of different cars of the same model is virtually identical, but there is a considerable variation in the size and shape of human beings of the same age and sex, even though all can be considered to be 'normal'. This huge range of normal variation is what defines human beings as individuals. Every human being differs from every other human being in some respect,

and there is a wide range of variation in all human structure and function – anatomical, physiological, biochemical, psychological and social. An important part of medical education is to gain an experience of the range of normal variation, partly so that you are able to decide whether or not a particular measurement or finding – for example a person's weight, the sounds that you hear over a patient's heart through your stethoscope, the results of a biochemical test or the way in which a patient behaves in relation to other people – falls within the accepted range of normal variation. If it does not, it may be one indication of disease or malfunction.

Second, unlike cars, human beings do have a 'mind of their own', and they must never be treated like inanimate objects. Finally, in the last resort, every component of a car can be disassembled and examined directly if necessary: with human beings, we are still mostly dependent on indirect evidence and fine judgement. In many respects, then, the car analogy is inaccurate, but we hope that it has served its limited purpose.

Problem-solving in practice

Although the GP makes use of all of the three main types of problem-solving process outlined above, he relies, perhaps more than the proponents of other specialties especially on hypothetico-deductive reasoning. This is partly because the business of dealing

with a large number of people whose initial complaints are completely undifferentiated demands some way of short-cutting through the painstaking intricacies of the inductive method, largely by cutting out lines of enquiry and examination that are likely to be unproductive. It is important to emphasise that an experienced doctor does this as a safe, discriminating and efficient modification of clinical method and as a process that, precisely because it arises from great skill and experience, may look deceptively simple to the observer.

You may have a chance to observe a GP consulting, even at a fairly early stage of your medical education. The frameworks in Table 1 and Figure 1 are given without any further detailed explanation. They are intended to be used as an aid to discussion with tutors, but remember that your tutor may have his or her own favourite alternative.

Clinical method

- This section introduces you to how doctors set about solving clinical problems, to help you understand this part of the clinical process when, for example, observing general practice consultations

- Highly experienced doctors tailor clinical method to individual circumstances whereas novices have to learn it in a very comprehensive and exhaustive way

- Experienced doctors therefore work more quickly, albeit still safely, mainly by cutting out lines of enquiry and examinations that they know are likely to be unproductive

Evidence-based medicine (EBM)

The phrase 'evidence-based medicine' was coined by a Canadian doctor, David Sackett, and his colleagues, to describe a way of practising medicine that involves the 'conscientious, explicit and judicious use of current best evidence in making decisions about the care of individual patients'. Its philosophical origins extend back to mid-19th century Paris and earlier. Critics of the EBM movement reckon that it is impractical in everyday practice and resent the implication that practising without EBM is practising poor medicine.

How to go about practising EBM

Several times each day every GP needs to find information to care for patients. Often this information is easily available: for example, look up a drug dose in the British National Formulary, use the practice directory to find out the time of the next Alcoholics Anonymous meeting, check the practice library for the European guidelines on the management of hypertension, phone a consultant colleague for information on a patient recently discharged from hospital.

Sometimes more detective work is required, particularly if you need information about the cause, diagnosis, prognosis or treatment of a clinical condition.

You are sitting in with a GP tutor and you see the following patients:

A six year old girl with a common fungal infection of the scalp (*tinea capitus*, common name ringworm) who lives with her mum, and three siblings, all under age 8 years. Mum is having difficulty coping, and is not the best at complying with medical advice. The GP mentions after the consultation that he is dubious about whether she will manage to apply a topical lotion to all her children and herself, and speculates that an oral treatment would be easier, and might be more effective if it were available.

A 56-year-old man who had a myocardial infarction last month was told in the hospital that he has heart failure. This sounds very scary to him, and he wants to know whether it will make any difference to how he will get on after the heart attack.

You could look up a textbook, or talk to your tutor, but this may not suffice.

Sackett has outlined the steps involved in using EBM in such situations (Box 1).

Box 1 The EBM steps

- Convert information needs into answerable questions
- Find the best evidence with which to answer the question
- Critically appraise the evidence for its validity (closeness to the truth) and usefulness
- Apply the evidence

Asking questions you can answer

Consider the two clinical scenarios already used as examples and jot down any questions you have about them. Asked in the right way a good question will direct you towards finding the information you require, whereas if you are too woolly you will find the question impossible to answer helpfully. Sackett suggests that there are several parts to any 'well-built' question.

Elements of a well-built clinical question

- Define the patient group and problem (e.g. primary school children with ringworm, or people who have had a first myocardial infarction).
- Decide what intervention or factor you are considering and what comparison, if any, is necessary (e.g. an oral treatment for ringworm compared to standard topical treatment, or how the presence of heart failure affects outcome from MI compared to those without heart failure).
- Specify the outcome you are interested in (e.g. proportion of children in whom ringworm are eradicated, or five-year survival after first MI).

Did your jottings have all the elements of a good question? Asking questions in this way takes a bit of practice, but makes the next step much easier.

Finding the best evidence to answer the question

The following are good starting points.

MEDLINE database

This is maintained by the National Library of Medicine in the USA, and is the best source of up-to-date evidence. You can access MEDLINE from home via several free web-sites: e.g. try *http://www.medscape.com/server-java/MedlineSearchForm*.

There are several software packages available for searching the database (for example OVID, Silver Platter) so you need to familiarise yourself with whatever is in use in your university library or hospital. Searching MEDLINE effectively is an important skill.

Other databases

There are many other specialist data bases, and the following are only a few of the most important at time of going to press:

The Cochrane Collaboration (http://www.cochrane.org/). The major product of the collaboration is the Cochrane Database of Systematic Reviews which is marketed as part of The Cochrane Library.

The ScHARR Guide (http://www.shef.ac.uk/uni/academic/R-/scharr/ir/netting.html). A comprehensive introduction to evidence-based practice on the internet.

Centre for EBM (http://www.eboncall.com) located in Oxford, UK.

Health Information Research Unit (http://hiru.hirunet.mcmaster.ca/). Evidence-Based Health Informatics at McMaster University, Hamilton, Canada.

NLM Clinical Trials Database (http://clinicaltrials.gov/). A consumer-friendly database by the National Institutes of Health, USA. It provides easy access to information about the location of clinical trials, their design and purpose, criteria for participation and additional disease and treatment information.

Healthfinder (http://www.healthfinder.gov/default.htm). A rich source of health information established by the US Government.

Bandolier (http://www.jr2.ox.ac.uk/bandolier/). A widely distributed UK journal on evidence-based health, including summaries of numbers needed to treat for many common interventions.

Appraising the evidence

Once you have found something which you think may fit the bill in terms of what information and evidence you need to help answer your question, you now need to decide whether you think it is up to scratch. What did the investigators do in their study? Did they do it right? Thus, is it valid? If the study is valid, what does it say (ie. what are the actual results)? Finally, will the results help you with the question you asked in the very first place, and will this help you with the management of your patient?

The quality of published papers

It is important to consider the following:

- Was the study original?
- Were the subjects recruited from a hospital population, from primary care or for some other more specialist group, such as prisoners or injecting drug users in the community. This will affect the relevance of results to other groups.
- Who was included (or more often excluded) from the study? People who have pre-existing illnesses, speak languages other than English, or who live in different cultures (e.g. travellers or refugees) are often left out of studies.
- Did the study happen in a real life situation, or was the study setting contrived, with new elements to the treatment programme? There are advantages to the contrived setting, in that the benefits from any intervention are likely to be greater, but it may limit the applicability of study to your own patients. Also, how accurately was the intervention described? Do you know **exactly** what the investigators did?
- Do you think the study design was rational? In particular, did the authors use a sensible intervention, did they compare it with something relevant (e.g. current best treatment is often a more helpful comparison than placebo)? What main outcome measure was used? While it might seem easier to measure symptoms (e.g. mood or pain) or ability to function (like how far a patient can walk or how well asthmatic children can play sport), in fact, good studies should measure outcomes which demonstrate a concrete end-point, such as longer life (e.g. improved five-year survival) or lower incidence of particular medical conditions, like myocardial infarction. Was the assessment of the outcome blind? That is, whoever is assessing the

outcome must be unaware of whether the patient was receiving the new treatment, or the comparison treatment. Otherwise it is possible or even probable that in their enthusiasm for the study, the investigator will over-estimate the benefit of the new intervention.

- Was systematic bias avoided, preferably by randomising patients to treatment and comparison groups, but otherwise by ensuring that groups compared to each other were as similar as possible? Did the investigators manage to ensure that nearly all of the study participants were followed up for the full period of the study? If not, bias in the results will creep in.
- Was the study large enough? The 'sample size' needs to be able to detect any effect that does exist. Was the period of follow-up long enough?

The hierarchy of studies – getting your bearings

There are a limited number of study designs:

- **Experiments** – when some strategy is carried out on volunteer (or animal) in laboratory or artificial conditions.
- **Clinical trials** – where a new treatment, compared to an existing or no treatment, is offered to a group of patients, whose progress is followed over time.
- **Surveys** – which may be postal or by interview, where a group of people are asked the same question, or have the same measurements taken for comparison purposes.
- **Observational studies** – of which cohort, case-control, cross-sectional studies and case reports are examples

Conventional evidence-based medicine wisdom states that there is a variation in the weight that should be applied to results according to the study design used by the investigators, as follows:

- systematic reviews and meta-analyses (reviews that use statistical

methods to combine the results of several similar trials)
- randomised controlled trials
- cohort studies
- case-control studies
- cross-sectional surveys
- case reports.

In essence there are five broad areas that you will commonly meet when reading papers. Each type of question is likely to require a different study design, as follows:

- therapy (surgical or medical): randomised controlled trial
- diagnosis : cross-sectional survey (comparing new test and existing gold-standard test)
- screening : cross-sectional survey
- prognosis : cohort study
- causation : case-control study.

Although it is important that all clinicians should be familiar with the concepts of formulating questions, searching for and appraising the evidence, it is in reality, too difficult for most of us. This is particularly so in general practice, where there is such a breadth of issues, problems and questions to contend with. In a random survey of 25% of GPs in the Wessex region of England, more than 90% of the GPs who replied welcomed EBM and agreed that its practice can improve patient care, but stated that learning evidence handling skills is not a priority. However, they were keen to and often do use evidence-based evaluations of studies generated by other sources. Probably the most useful summary evidence is that provided by 'Clinical Evidence' which is a regularly updated compilation of summaries, designed to answer common and important questions that arise every day in clinical practice.

To get good at EBM you will need to formulate good clinical questions during your attachments, practice your critical appraisal skills and read around the literature. You will, however, be constantly surprised at the lack of evidence for common practices in medicine.

Evidence-based medicine

- Evidence-based medicine has been around for a long time.
- Starting with a good question helps in finding good evidence.
- Getting to know your way around a few databases is important.
- It helps to be familiar with research methodology.
- Appraising the evidence requires time and skills.

Inequalities in health

There is now compelling international evidence to show that people who live in disadvantaged circumstances have more illness, disability and stress, and a shorter life, than those who are better off. 'Equity' and 'equality' are terms that are often used interchangeably, but there is a difference in their definitions. *Equity* is taken to relate to the distribution of the available resources over the population on the basis of need and an equitable sharing of the cost of providing such services. *Equality* in health is a step beyond equity, guaranteeing an equitable distribution of the available health services; it implies that each individual is offered the same opportunity to enjoy good health.

In most health-care systems, issues of equity, which are really about fairness, emerge very quickly. In 1971, Tudor Hart proposed the inverse care law to highlight the fact that 'the quality of medical care, and particularly GP care, is lowest where the needs of the population are highest'.

The main determinants of health can be broadly grouped into two categories (Fig. 1):

1. *Fixed factors* such as age, gender and hereditary, about which little can be done
2. *Modifiable factors* such as individual life-style factors, social and community influences, living and working conditions, and finally general socio-economic cultural and environmental conditions.

The health-care responses when tackling inequalities in health have fallen into the following categories:

- strengthening individuals
- strengthening communities
- improving access to essential facilities and services.

Strengthening individuals is based on the premise that building up people's knowledge, motivation and skills will enable them to alter their personal risk factors and cope better with the stresses and strains of outside influences. The focus on strengthening communities lies on how people can work together for mutual support and how they can influence the health hazards in their own community. The government sector is increasingly recognising the strengths of individuals, families and voluntary organisations in creating healthier living conditions (Table 1).

Most industrialised countries have made enormous strides in improving housing and utilities, increasing the age of early school-leaving and optimising family planning services. Access to good-quality, free health care at the point of use is still, however, a major issue for many health-care systems, the UK's National Health Service (NHS) being an honourable exception.

Table 1 **Communities working together**

- Reduction of substance abuse
- Socialisation of young people into the community
- Improving access to formal and informal health care
- Crèche and pre-school facilities

Primary care

The Acheson Report (1998) has pointed out that access to effective primary care is influenced by the geographical distribution and availability of primary care staff. In Dublin, for example, the most deprived areas may not have a local practice in their area, whereas the more salubrious areas are 'over-doctored' (Fig. 2).

People living in poorer areas are likely to experience difficulty in finding a doctor out of hours and are more likely to be served by a single-handed practitioner working from poor premises. Those communities at greatest risk of ill-health tend to experience the least satisfactory access to a full range of preventive services and a poorer uptake of such services. Health promotion claims by GPs in the NHS are highest in the least deprived, and lowest in the most deprived, areas (Acheson Report 1998). GP referral rates are higher for patients from deprived areas for both physical and psychiatric illnesses.

Once patients enter the hospital service, there is evidence of an inequity in referral onwards to investigations for specialist cardiac services for the deprived. In the NHS, the mortality from coronary heart disease in South Asians is, for example, 40% higher than that of the general population, but the rates of coronary artery bypass grafting and angioplasty in this subgroup are below the national average.

The use of alcohol, drugs and tobacco is influenced by the wider social setting. Smoking and alcohol are a disproportionate drain on the income of the less well-off. In a low income household, over 4% of the income may be spent on tobacco compared with 0.8% of the family income in a well-off household with a smoker. Drugs, alcohol and tobacco may provide a temporary release from stress and reality, but alcohol dependence leads to further downward social mobility, and tobacco is a major cause of ill-health and premature death (Figs 3 and 4).

Although health-care provision is not the most important aspect of tackling inequality in health, it can nonetheless make a difference (Table 2). Patients from socio-economically deprived areas have a higher consultation rate for illness. They also

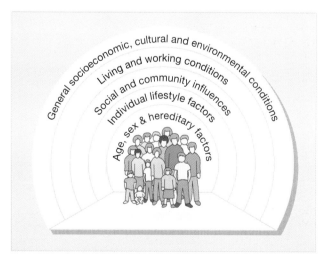

Fig. 1 **The main determinants of health.** Source: Dahlgren and Whitehead (1991).

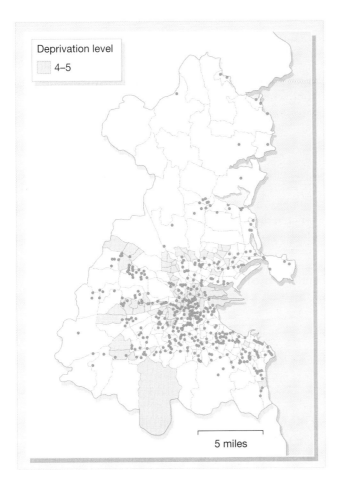

Fig. 2 **Areas of high deprivation (levels 4–5) and surgery location in the Dublin area.**

women, in their take-up of family planning services and cervical screening. Practices with a female doctor and/or nurse are more likely to reach cervical cytology targets in the NHS, but access to female GPs is poor in areas with a high concentration of Asian residents. A number of interventions and initiatives have thus been carried out among socio-economically deprived populations (Table 3).

There is no evidence of any unwillingness to contemplate changes to health behaviour among the socio-economically deprived, but significant barriers, including those of time, space and income, exist for low-income families. Information is often not readily available, and there may be a lack of lay support for the adoption of positive health strategies. In general, for example, people know that smoking is bad for them, but those with little control over their lives continue to smoke in order to cope with the stresses of their existence (Table 4).

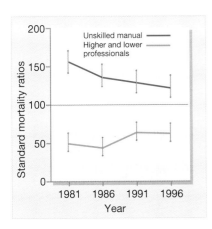

Fig. 3 **Trends in mortality by occupational class for men aged 15–64 years (1981–1996).**

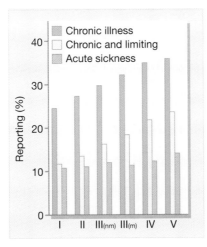

Fig. 4 **Morbidity in Great Britain by socio-economic group, 1991.** Source: Office of Population Censuses and Surveys (1993).

tend to experience the least satisfactory access to preventive services, including cancer screening programmes, health promotion and immunisation. A lack of access to female GPs can be a deterrent to women in general, especially to very young and Asian

Table 3 **Characteristics of effective intervention among socio-economically deprived patients**

- Intervenes at an individual level
- Recognses the need for information, understanding and skills
- Takes on board the limited room for manoeuvre of the deprived patient
- Combines practical advice with training
- Loan of safety equipment: fire and stairguards, baby seats for cars, use of trained lay people, e.g. community mothers scheme (Johnson et al 1993)

Table 4 **Social determinants of health**

- People fall into long-term disadvantage
- The social and psychological environment affects health
- A good environment in early childhood is vital
- Work impacts on health
- Unemployment and job insecurity impact on health
- Friendship and social cohesion have positive effects on health
- Social exclusion is dangerous to health
- Alcohol, nicotine and illicit drugs are markers of social deprivation
- High-quality fresh food is essential to good health
- Healthy transport means more walking, cycling and better public transport

Source: World Health Organization (1998)

Table 2 **Access to effective primary care**

- Geographical distribution of staff
- Availability of staff
- Range and quality of facilities
- Training and education of staff
- Recruitment of primary care staff
- Cultural training and sensitivity
- Organisation of services, timing of services and location of services 'around the corner'
- Availbility of affordable and safe transport

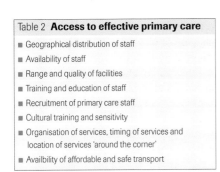

Inequalities in health

- People who live in disadvantaged circumstances have more illness, disability and higher mortality than the better-off.

- Poorer areas are often 'under doctored' compared to better off areas.

- People from deprived areas have poorer access to preventative services including immunisation.

- People now know smoking is bad for them but the less well-off smoke in order to cope with stressful lives.

Family medicine

In the UK, GPs are (or used to be) commonly known as 'family doctors', and the term 'family practitioner' has been widely adopted in the USA by many primary care generalists. The family doctor concept is most likely to have applied primarily to rural areas, where there might only have been one single-handed doctor. In areas of larger population, and in modern times when single-handed practice is much less common, the model may be considerably diluted. It depends to an extent upon all members of a family being registered with the same practice, but this is quite commonly not the case, mainly because, on marriage or co-habitation, partners frequently choose to stay with their original GP.

Of all doctors, however, GPs are usually the most aware of family and environmental influences on health and are often best placed to deal with them. Family structures, or their equivalent, are generally the building blocks of all civilised societies. It is important to emphasise that, when they work successfully, family structures provide invaluable nurture and support for their members, both in sickness and in health. When, however, family dynamics go wrong, the family may contribute to the development of ill-health.

Families go through a predictable life cycle (Fig. 1), each stage having its own potential problems. Some of these are discussed later in the book (see Sections on age related and sex related problems).

How the family and environment may cause ill-health

Upbringing

How we are nurtured and moulded by our parents is perhaps one of the most important ways in which family relationships may affect our subsequent health (Box 1). The relationships in some family groups may be frankly abusive, either physically and/or mentally, and although we do not deal with such extremes in detail here, GPs are constantly on the alert for possible criminal abuse (Box 2), which may take place in apparently stable and 'nice' families, including those of professionals such as doctors themselves.

Nature or nurture?

It is difficult to separate the effects of inheritance and upbringing. Genetics research (see pp 94–95) is increasingly uncovering predispositions to disease

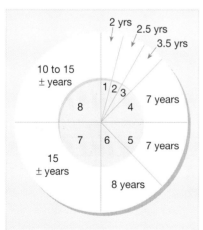

1. Newly married
   (without children)
2. Birth of first child
   (oldest child, birth – 30 months)
3. Families with preschool children
   (oldest child, 30 months – 6 years)
4. Children in school
   (oldest child, 6–13 years)
5. Families with teenagers
   (oldest child, 13–20 years)
6. Launching years
   (first to last child leaving home)
7. Parents alone
   (last child gone – retirement)
8. Retirement and later years
   (retirement – death of both spouses)

Fig. 1 **The family life cycle.** Source: McWhinney (1981). Modified from Duvall (1977).

Box 1 Parent behaviours that are potentially damaging

- One or both parents being persistently unresponsive to a child's care-eliciting behaviour, or being actively disparaging and rejecting
- Discontinuities of parenting, occurring more or less frequently, including periods in a hospital or institution
- Persistent threats by parents not to love a child, used as a means of controlling him or her
- Threats by parents to abandon the family, used either as a method of disciplining the child or as a way of coercing the spouse
- Threats by one parent either to desert or even to kill the other, or else to commit suicide (each of these being more common than might be supposed)
- Inducing a child to feel guilty by claiming that his behaviour is or will be responsible for the parent's illness or death.

Source: Bowlby (1969). Quoted in Henderson A S (1988)

Box 2 Maltreatment of children

- Non-accidental injury. This may be suspected when children show unusual, difficult to account for, injuries, for example bite marks, cigarette burns or scalds, or bone or periosteal injuries, or display indications of multiple injury over time, such as bruises of different ages. Shaking a young child is a particularly dangerous form of abuse that can result in serious brain injury. Parents have often had a troubled or abusive childhood themselves; the child may be difficult to manage or may be emotionally rejected by the parents; there are often underlying marital problems, particularly with very young parents; and there may be a lack of a supporting family and social structure for the parents.
- Sexual abuse. Although associated with interference by 'strangers', sexual abuse is actually more likely to be carried out by family members or friends of the family.
- Child neglect. Children may be harmed by negligence or a lack of 'common sense', particularly when the parents are themselves of low intelligence, are poorly educated and have poor role modelling from their own deprived childhood.
- Emotional abuse and deprivation. A child may be well looked after physically but suffer from a withdrawal of affection, insecurity and a general atmosphere in the household of repression and hostility. These subtle forms of abuse may be difficult to detect (see Box 1)
- Munchausen syndrome by proxy is a well-publicised but rare and bizarre form of abuse in which illness in the child is falsely created by a carer, usually the mother. See also Hull and Johnston (1993)

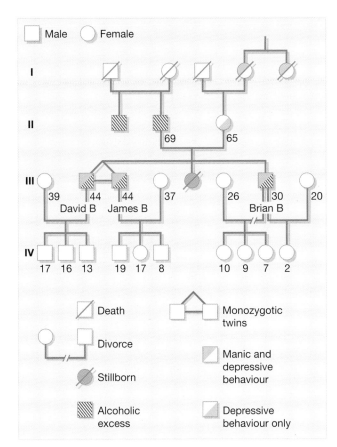

Fig. 2 **The inheritance pattern of bipolar affective disorder in a family.** ○ = female; □ = male Source: Rakel (1977).

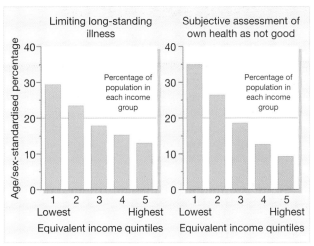

Fig. 3 **Age/sex-standardised number of individuals reporting morbidity in each equivalent income group as a percentage of all individuals reporting morbidity.** Source: General Household Survey, (1985), *from Benzeval et al (1995).*

that are wholly or partially determined by inheritance. GPs are often struck by how patterns of ill-health 'run in families', and the use of family charts (Fig. 2) may help in breaking, or at least anticipating, these patterns. In the example given (bipolar affective disorder, a type of depressive illness), there are probably both genetic and environmental factors.

Family circumstances

The social standing of the parents, cultural (including religious) and other social attitudes, and the economic circumstances of the family all have a potential effect on causing, or conversely combatting, ill-health. Of these, the most pervasive effects are those of socio-economic deprivation.

It might be thought that, compared with the devastating poverty of so-called 'Third World' countries, few people in the developed world can be considered to be deprived. Within developed countries, however, it has been very convincingly shown that although the basics of life (shelter, food, clothing etc) may have been well met, and there may even be luxury items such as televisions and cars, families that are poor in relation to others in that country ('relative deprivation') consistently experience

much poorer health. In Britain, people in the lowest fifth of the population in terms of income are four times more likely to report their health as being not good as are those in the highest fifth (Fig. 3). Although it is difficult to separate out the effect of a difference in life-style (smoking, alcohol consumption, exercise etc), unemployment, lone parenthood and low wages are thought to be major factors in a vicious circle of poverty, resulting in 'social exclusion', stress and anxiety, and a limitation of life choices, as well as militating against possible desirable changes in life-style.

The role of primary health care

The main role of primary health-care staff is to be alert to the possibility of family problems. Teamwork, usually involving health visitors, social work staff and community nurses, as well as the doctor, is particularly essential in tackling simple family problems. Good communication between members of the team is also essential, and visits to the family home and/or simple family therapy with couples or family groups may be part of the team's strategy. For more major problems, it is usually desirable to seek help from specialist family therapists (Box 3).

Box 3 Psychosocial problems likely to benefit from behavioural family therapy strategies

- Children's conduct disorders
- Learning disabilities and autism
- Adolescent behavioural disturbance
- Marital and family conflict
- Sexual dysfunction
- Drug and alcohol misuse
- Family violence and child abuse
- Pre-marital counselling
- Divorce mediation
- Eating disorders
- Suicide prevention
- Residential care: homes, hostels, etc
- Criminal offending problems

Adapted from Falloon et al (1993)

Family medicine

- The idyllic model of the GP as 'family doctor' may never have been universally true and is now considerably diluted, especially in urban practice.

- However, modern general practice training lays great emphasis on family and environmental influences on health, even if an individual GP may now less frequently look after all family members.

- Families have both bad and good influences on health of individuals and these influences vary at different stages in the life cycle of a family.

- The effects of genetic inheritance and upbringing are difficult to separate but the most pervasive influence is adverse socio-economic circumstances.

- Tackling family problems usually needs a team approach, with specialist input for major difficulties.

Changes in society

Society is continuously changing; indeed, some argue that this is its main characteristic. Changes take place around us all the time in a range of different areas – technological, cultural, political, social, economic and demographic. Some of these are, of course, related. One way of studying such development in society is by the work of the National Centre for Social Research, which publishes the annual *British Social Attitudes Reports*.

A number of social issues are used to highlight the kind of attitudinal and behavioural alterations that have taken place over the past decades. The social and cultural changes addressed here focus on the role and position of GPs, although some wider issues such as the changing family, social exclusion, increases in leisure and the role of the media are also covered. This chapter concludes with two examples of societal change in:

- the use of so-called 'illegal drugs', or 'drug misuse'
- sexual behaviour and attitudes towards sex.

Changes in society: the importance for GP

GPs, more than hospital doctors, have to deal with people living in their own community. They have to be aware of the circumstances and conditions in which people live and the types of alteration taking place in the lives of their patients. Some of these are personal: people are becoming older, getting married or getting divorced, having children, moving house and so on. We can also recognise some collective social changes: more people, for example, are getting divorced than did 20 years ago, more women have their first child at a later age, and more young people in Britain than ever before are attending university. What is important is that each individual is not an isolated person but forms part of the wider society. It is necessary to consider people's altering socio-economic environment in order to have a better understanding of their health and their health-related behaviour. Being aware of this can help the doctor to understand problems from a patient's perspective, which can be helpful in determining the best intervention for that particular patient.

At the same time, the work experience of GPs has also been modified. Working practice has, for example, altered so that there are far fewer single-handedly run GP practices and an increase in the number of larger group practices. The latter often include a range of other health-care providers such as practice (or treatment room) nurses, community midwives, health visitors or community psychiatric nurses. GPs' expectations of life-style and workload, with a greater emphasis on their private life and family expectations, have influenced general practice in these areas.

Patients have become more demanding as a part of a general increase in so-called 'consumerism'. Health can be seen as a commodity that responds to consumer demands. Thus, on the one hand, we see a growth in the number of health-food shops, exercise videos and low-calorie drinks; on the other hand, GPs experience more demanding patients in their surgeries. A consumer demand for immediate service, rather than a GP appointment in 4 days time, has led to the introduction of NHS Direct, a telephone health help line run by the National Health Service.

The changing family

The composition of the family is now more varied – more children are born out of wedlock, the so-called nuclear family is in decline, and more people are living alone. Since the 1960s, the number of babies born outside marriage has risen from under 10% to nearly 40% of all births at the end of the 20th century (Hall 2000). There are now more single-parent families and more families 'headed' by women as a result of the higher divorce rate. Since many divorced people remarry or establish new long-term relationships, their children may have multiple sets of parents or siblings with different surnames. If, for example, the children stay with their mother after the divorce and she remarries, these children gain a second father (with perhaps an extra set of siblings and/or grandparents). If their natural father establishes a long-term relationship with another woman, the children may similarly gain new relations.

Culture and the structure of society

Our multi-ethnic culture is constantly changing. Immigration into the UK in the 19th century consisted largely of poor Irish, whereas at the end of the 19th century and in the early 20th century, the largest group was Eastern European Jews. In the second half of the 20th century, most immigrants into the UK came from ex-colonies in the Third World, such as the West Indies and the Indian subcontinent. Many immigrants ended up living and working in the big cities.

Deprivation and social exculsion

From the beginning to the end of the 20th century, the real national income per head of population quadrupled in the UK. As a result the standard of living rose. All groups in society were 'better-off' in 2000 than in 1900, but the lowest socio-economic groups did not benefit as much from this economic growth as did the rest. There are continuous concerns about poorer people's access to health care: from the range of services used, the timing of the first contact and the uptake of health promotion messages to the appropriateness of the available health services for different populations.

Changes in leisure

Many people have more time and money available for leisure. We work on average fewer hours per week than our grandparents, even though a 1998 survey revealed that full-time employees in the UK worked on average the longest hours in Europe, namely 45.7 hours per week for men and 40.7 for women (Hall 2000).

Despite this, most of us have more time available for leisure than previous generations did. In our spare time we watch more television than our parents and have a more sedentary life-style. We take more holidays, and when we go away, we are more likely to travel further and more likely to go abroad. Consequently, we have more experience of other cultures, universal events and or universal culture.

The role of the media

One of the main changes over the past century has been the growth of the media, involving a rapid and ever-continuing development from radio and cinema to terrestrial television, then to commercial and satellite television, and more recently to computers and the Internet.

Television programmes such as *ER*, an American television series about the 'emergency room' of a large hospital, gives people experiences and expectations of health, and this can have a knock-on effect: more people, for example, than the number officially trained have carried out resuscitation in Scotland, which the Scottish Ambulance Service believes is due to people picking up the technique from TV programmes and films. One of the risks with this is, of course, that people 'think' they know what to do but do not in fact, causing more harm than good. On a more morbid note, our children will have seen more deaths on television by the time they are 15 than our grandparents will have seen in a lifetime.

The Internet is only just beginning to make an impact on people's life being used for information, recreation and shopping. It is claimed that after 'sex', health-related terms are the most often used search words on the Internet, and doctors now regularly report that patients come to consultations with information gleaned from the Internet.

Examples of changes in society

The social behaviour related to, and attitudes towards, illegal drug use and sexual behaviour are investigated below in more detail.

Drug misuse in society

Drugs derived from natural sources, rather than those synthetically produced, have been used for medical and recreational purposes for thousands of years. For example, only since 1971 have British doctors been barred, under the Misuse of Drugs Act, from prescribing cannabis.

If we consider changes over the past three decades, we see, for example, that smoking, and similarly drinking and driving (Box 1), is becoming less acceptable in many industrialised societies, with the introduction of bans on smoking in public places, legislation against tobacco advertising on television etc. At the same time, we see a relaxation in attitude towards so-called soft drugs (cannabis, hashish or marijuana) in many countries. In the UK, there are regular calls for the decriminalisation of cannabis, the police sometimes ignoring the

---

| Box 1 **Drinking and driving is becoming less socially acceptable** |

Surveys indicate that attitudes towards drinking and driving are slowly changing. More people agree that the police should have the power to take random breath tests. In 1968, 25% of people in Britain approved of random breath testing, the corresponding figure being 48% in 1975 and 78% in 1988. Research has also found that a larger proportion of the population now approves of tougher penalties for drink-driving offenders than did 30 years ago.

| Box 2 **General practitioners and drug misusing patients** |

Doctors need to be:

- aware that it occurs
- prepared to enquire about all forms of non-prescribed drug use, both legal and illegal
- sensitive to patient's views
- non-judgemental and (in general) highly confident when dealing with illegal drug use
- evidence-based and dispassionate in discussing the potential for harmful effects, recognising that illegal drug users can be ill informed
- prepared to offer useful and realistic support and treatment to hose who recognise their addiction
- alert to the widespread problems of manipulation and abuse of GP prescribing by drug misusers and have systems in place to minimise this
- aware that drug misuse is frequently symptomatic of underlying social and psychological difficulties, indicating the need for a holistic approach to management.

---

possession of small amounts for personal use. Calls for legalisation arise from a wide spectrum of society, including representatives of the police, politicians and the judiciary. Also more references are made to the use of soft drugs in the media.

But what does such social change mean for the doctor (Box 2)? First, the new generation of doctors are more likely to have tried soft drugs than are their older counterparts. Second, observing the softening attitudes towards drug misuse does not, however, mean that doctors need to condone it.

Sexual behaviour

A second example is the changing attitude towards sexual health, in particular towards intercourse before the age of 16. The 1960s are often seen as the period when attitudes towards

sex became more open, but it did not stop there. The proportion of young people, especially girls (Todd et al 1999), who have sexual intercourse before the age of 16 is, for example, still increasing (Johnson et al 1994), even though surveys also report that young people often regret having had sexual intercourse this young (Dickson et al 1998, Wight et al 2000).

Changing sexual behaviour requires a revamping of sexual health education, and society's attitudes towards health promotion are also advancing. What is possible in terms of sexual health education in the early 21st century was simply not socially acceptable before the late 1980s, when the threat of HIV became 'real': in 1982 one could not speak about or advertise condoms in the same open way as one can in 2002, which is definitely a step in the right direction.

| *Changes in society* |

- Society is changing all the time. Some of this, such as certain technological advances allowing the mass introduction of the mobile telephone, is happening rapidly, some, however, occurs more gradually, for example in our attitudes towards race and ethnicity, or marriage.

- The changing mores in society have implications for health policies.

- Doctors need to be aware of this in order to be able to deliver the most appropriate kind of health services.

Risks and health

Risk factors

Over recent years, people have become increasingly aware that risk can be established for many disorders, such as congenital anomalies and cardiac disease. Consequently, risk factor identification has become a major industry in research: 80 000 papers on risk were published between 1987 and 1991, and 300 risk factors have been identified for coronary artery disease alone. Some of this research is driven by powerful statistical packages, the findings revealing associations that are both clinically unimportant and unhelpful. The data used in establishing risks generally derive from populations, which poses problems when attempts are made to translate these to the individual. The populations sometimes also comprise healthy people, which makes it even more difficult to extrapolate to a single sick patient.

It is, however, important to be aware of risks as some of these can be modified by the patient or the doctor. Equally, some risks cannot be modified, the individual patient currently having little control over these personal risk factors: a patient with a strong family history of schizophrenia, for example, is vulnerable to the illness no matter what he or she does. Similarly, the genetic make-up of the parents will determine whether their child has cystic fibrosis, and a woman with a strong close family history of breast cancer has a high risk of developing the illness.

Other risks are modifiable with good information and effort. Smokers who stop lower their risk of lung cancer and heart disease. Patients who reduce their weight and sugar intake decrease their risk of type II diabetes. Parents who fully vaccinate their children all but remove their risk of developing disabling childhood illnesses.

Knowledge, attitudes and practice, and the KA–P gap

When discussing risk, it is helpful to break it up into knowledge, attitudes and practice. A population or a patient may have knowledge about the risk inherent in a particular health practice such as cigarette-smoking or safe drinking, but this knowledge may be disregarded on grounds such as 'it does not apply to me' or 'it is my body and I will do as I want'. Patients may alternatively have a positive attitude and want to limit their risk, thus seeking help from their doctor. This group includes a large number of reasonable people, but it is the group that often has trouble putting advice into practice. There is a large gap – known as 'the KA–P gap' – between knowledge, positive attitudes and practice.

There are many barriers to modifying risk, such as life-style, personality and health beliefs, but having control over one's life is probably a much underrated factor in modifying risk. For example, a middle-aged man who smokes and is over-weight may have to work long hours to make ends meet, having little or no time for exercise, being aware that tobacco is bad for him but believing he needs it to cope. Doctors who are evangelical about modifying risk often find that exploring the barriers to change allows them to set realistic targets for their patients within a supportive framework.

Risk

Relative risk is the ratio of risk of an event, disease or death among those exposed, to the risk in those who are not exposed. It is increasingly being used synonymously with 'odds ratio'. In the Veterans Administration (VA) Study (Table 1) the relative risk reduction in patients with target organ damage on entry into the trial was 62%, whereas in those without target organ damage, the relative risk reduction was 59%. However, this does not convey the yield or efficiency of a treatment.

The number-needed-to-treat (NNT) is the number of patients who must be treated to prevent an adverse event. This concept gets across the yield or efficiency of a treatment in a manner that relative risk does not. In the VA Study (Table 1), the NNT in order to prevent one adverse event in those with target organ damage is 7 while it is 17 in those without target organ damage. Students are often surprised by this method of expressing information but it leads to interesting discussions with patients, as well as to informed decisions.

Risks and health

Measuring benefits and risks in medicine (Table 2) can be divided into the following categories:

- the consequences of doing nothing (the patient's risk of illness if there is no intervention)
- the risk of harm from the procedure or treatment itself
- patients who are at high risk of illness and for whom a treatment exists to reduce that risk
- a comparison of the outcomes of different approaches to the prevention, diagnosis and treatment of conditions.

Table 1 Measure of efficacy of antihypertensives and placebo in the 3 year Veterans Administration study

Patient condition at entry to study	Rates of adverse events[1]		Relative risk reduction (%)	Absolute risk reduction	Number-needed-to-treat to prevent one adverse event[1]
	Placebo (%)	Treatment (%)			
Target organ damage	22	8.5	62	0.137	7
No target organ damage	9.8	4.0	59	0.098	17

[1]Sudden death, stroke, myocardial infarction, congestive cardiac failure, hypertension and dissecting aneurysum
After Laupacis et al (1988)

Table 2 Relationship of risk factors to health

Risk	Impact on health
Socio-economic	Strong links between poverty and ill-health
Environmental	Pollution, asthma, eczema
Genetic/family	Cystic fibrosis, schizophrenia, heart disease, diabetes
Occupational	Deafness, eczema/dermatitis, stress
Life-style	Alcohol, drugs, sexually transmitted diseases, diet
Travel	Communicable diseases
Behavioural	Risk-taking: bicycle helmets, unprotected sex
Poor education	Poor health practices in both the developed and the underdeveloped world
Illness	Psychiatric illness predisposes to suicide. Hyperlipidaema predisposes to myocardial infarction and hypertension to strokes
Cultural	Tolerance of alcohol: 'boys will be boys'. Resistance to genetic screening in Catholic and Muslim countries

---

Box 1   Explanation of treatment to a mild hypertensive male

If 100 men like you are followed for five years, about two will have a stroke, 98 will not. We do not know whether you are one of the two or one of the 98. If you reduce your blood pressure by taking antihypertensive medication, you will jump to another group. Then out of 100 men like you, one will have a stroke, 99 will not. We do not know whether you are the one or one of the 99. Which group do you wish to belong to: those who accept the status quo or those who take medication?

This explanation does not, however, address side-effects among the treated group, which are always much higher than is expected: if 100 men are treated with a thiazide diuretic for hypertension, 8 will have an abnormal glucose tolerance test, 10 will experience erectile difficulties and 4 will develop gout. Other antihypertensive medications produce a different side-effect profile, but the overall incidence of side-effects remains remarkably similar despite what the promotional literature says.

Multiple factors impact on health, surprisingly few, however, being influenced by direct clinical intervention. Those which are amenable to clinical intervention need:

- the education of both medical staff and patients about proven benefits, as with successful breast-feeding programmes
- enquiry approach – merely asking patients about alcohol consumption makes a difference to their intake
- practical help such as information leaflets, medication and medical support, smoking being a good example here.

Altering risk factors

Harm reduction is emerging as a more realistic approach whereby the risk to self and others is reduced, albeit not abolished. This approach often makes demands on society's simplistic approach to prevention but is pragmatic. The following are examples of this approach:

- the use of bicycle helmets to reduce head injury in case of road traffic accidents
- no smoking areas in restaurants, pubs, home and office in order to reduce the impact of passive smoking
- the provision of water at rave parties to reduce the dehydrating effects of ecstasy
- methadone programmes to reduce the health and social risks associated with intravenous drug use.

Explaining risks to patients

This is surprisingly complex because many people have difficulty understanding both the concept and the statistics involved. The concept is important because it requires patients to understand that people like them, but not them as individuals, are at risk: the patient understandably wants to know whether he or she will be the one who is at risk. A number of graphical methods, such as the European Cardiac Society's chart to explain risk in heart disease, can help here.

Several models of explaining risk are used; these can be summarised as follows:

- *Probability*: 'your chances of developing the illness are 1 in 100'
- *Actuarial*: 'men in your age bracket who continue to smoke lose 5 years of life, based on an average life expectancy of 72 years' (see also Box 1)
- *Analogy*: 'the chances of your developing a brain tumour are about the same as being knocked down by a bus'
- *Comparative*: 'the risk of your developing diabetes, given your age, build and family history, is about the same as your sister's'.

Recent trials

The following important trials are summarised using NNT formats:

The West of Scotland Coronary Prevention Study (WOSCOPS) was a primary prevention trial of over 6500 men using pravastatin that reduced the risk of non-fatal myocardial infarction (MI) by 31% and the overall mortality by 22%. The results suggest that treatment of 1000 such patients with pravastatin 40 mg daily for 5 years will prevent seven deaths from cardiovascular causes and 20 non-fatal MI.

The Scandinavian Simvastatin Survival Study (4S) is a secondary prevention study of over 4000 patients with previous MI or angina and a cholesterol concentration of 5.5–8.0 mmol/L. It produced a 42% reduction in the risk of death from coronary heart disease (CHD). This study suggests that treating 100 patients with simvastatin 20–40 mg daily for 6 years will prevent 4 deaths from CHD and 7 non-fatal MIs.

The Cholesterol and Recurrent Events trial (CARE) is a secondary prevention trial of over 4000 patients (mostly men) with a past history of MI and a cholesterol concentration of less than 6.2 mmol/L. The study reduced deaths from CHD or non-fatal MI by 24%, lessened the need for coronary artery bypass grafting or angioplasty by 27% and decreased the risk of developing a stroke by 31%. The study suggests that treating 100 patients with pravastatin 40 mg daily for 5 years will prevent 11 deaths from CHD and 26 non-fatal MIs.

The recent LIPID study is a secondary prevention study of over 9000 patients with a history of MI or unstable angina and an initial plasma cholesterol level of 4–7 mmol/L. The study showed that 40 mg pravastatin reduced all cardiovascular events by 29% and death from CHD by 24%. In order to prevent one death from CHD over a 6 year period, 52 high-risk patients would need to be treated.

Risks and health

- Risk data comes from population studies whereas patients want to know 'Am I at risk?'
- Some risks can be modified by both doctor and patient.
- Having control over one's life is a much underrated factor in health.
- Harm reduction is a pragmatic approach to risk reduction.
- Explaining risk is difficult but models do exist.

General principles

Most people can expect to live longer than did previous generations. One hundred years ago, men lived to 45 and women to 50 years, although if they survived the first year, the life expectancy overall increased by 5 years for both men and women. Today the picture is totally different in the Western world, men living into their early 70s and women to their late 70s, as a result of a variety of complex factors such as housing, diet, education and, probably least of all, medicine. Where medicine is concerned, it is the preventive aspects of medicine that have played a bigger part than the curative aspects in prolonging life expectancy.

The major infectious scourges of the 19th century were water-borne (cholera and enteric fever), occurred in childhood (diphtheria, measles, pertussis and scarlet fever) or were seen in young people (tuberculosis and polio). A modern-day medical student can expect to complete the course seeing only occasional cases of childhood or young people's infectious diseases. Other infectious diseases have of course taken their place, but the emphasis is still on prevention rather than cure.

Criteria for screening

Given the successes of childhood vaccination, preventing or merely arresting the development of disease is an attractive proposition, all the more so if the disease is disabling or fatal. This has provided an impetus for screening for such diseases. It is, however, not that straightforward, and every new screening test or procedure has to be viewed sceptically. The following, now widely accepted, criteria have been developed for the guidance of health-care planners and doctors:

1. The disease in question should be a serious health problem.
2. There should be a pre-symptomatic phase during which treatment can change the course of the disease more successfully than during the symptomatic phase.
3. The screening procedure and ensuing treatment should be acceptable to the public.
4. The screening procedure should have acceptable sensitivity (i.e. it should correctly identify those with the disease) and specificity (i.e. it

should correctly identify those without the disease).
5. The screening procedure and ensuing treatment should be cost-effective.

Prevention of ill-health

This can be defined as measures to reduce the risk of disease, illness, disability or any unwanted state of health, for example screening for breast and cervical problems. Prevention is usually divided into primary, secondary and tertiary prevention. Primary care provides an opportunity for all three stages of prevention, at both an individual and a community level.

Primary prevention

This increases the patient's ability to remain free of disease. Examples of primary prevention include the following:

- The prevalence of phenylketonuria is about 7 per 100 000 newborn babies, the condition thus being extremely rare. It can, however be diagnosed early and effectively by a heel prick test, and the associated mental retardation can be prevented by starting the appropriate diet on diagnosis.
- Immunisation against infectious diseases in childhood. The list of immunisations gets longer all the time as more acceptable and effective vaccines become available.
- The fluoridation of water helps to prevent dental caries.
- Life-style advice can prevent sun-induced skin cancer, alcohol problems, the diseases of smoking and sexually transmitted diseases.

There is inevitably an overlap between health promotion and prevention, as these examples show.

Secondary prevention

This involves the early detection of disease so that intervention may occur to delay its progression. Examples of secondary prevention are:

- the early detection of hypertension through systematic or opportunistic blood pressure recording; this allows advice, and if necessary treatment, to be provided during the pre-symptomatic phase of the illness
- the recognition of diabetes mellitus

by the detection of sugar in the urine in both pregnant and non-pregnant adults; such detection can be targetted at vulnerable groups such as pregnant women, older people and Asians in Britain.

Tertiary prevention

This is the management of established disease in order to minimise complications and disability. Several examples of tertiary prevention show this:

- Giving an aspirin to a patient immediately after a myocardial infarction reduces the risk of recurrence and improves mortality. The GP is well placed to do this when he or she is the professional first in contact with the patient.
- The blindness of diabetes can be prevented through good disease control, regular fundoscopy and prompt referral for the treatment of retinopathy.
- Rehabilitation following a stroke may restore some or the whole of the patient's previous life-style.

Opportunities for prevention in general practice

GPs are well placed to implement prevention. On average, GPs will see a particular patient 3–4 times per year, with the exception of young to middle-aged adult males, who may not consult at all.

The Royal College of General Practitioners has identified the seven most important opportunities for prevention as:

- family planning
- antenatal care
- immunisation
- fostering the bonds between mother and child
- discouraging smoking
- detecting and managing of raised blood pressure
- helping the bereaved.

Implementing opportunities for prevention

This can be done by screening or case-finding, as well as opportunistically.

Screening The practice may assist in a national or local screening campaign either by carrying out the procedure or by encouraging patients to avail themselves of opportunities. This may, for example, occur if a campaign is being organised to detect cancer of the cervix, breast cancer or glaucoma.

Case-finding   A family's interest may be triggered by a recent illness in one of their relatives. A myocardial infarction in a young man will often prompt other members of the family to come along for a cardiovascular work-up, including blood pressure monitoring and the measurement of lipid levels. It is not unusual for the doctor then to find that other members of the family are at risk of cardiovascular events.

Opportunistic   Fifty per cent of GP consultations are for minor, self-limiting illnesses, and such consultations may present an opportunity for a wider discussion of health. The doctor giving advice to a patient about an upper respiratory tract infection may, for example, take the opportunity to advise about smoking. Similarly, a young female patient presenting with acne may benefit from information on contraception.

Prevention – who pays?

There is now a general acceptance in medicine that selected preventive services and both secondary and tertiary prevention are worthwhile and indeed likely to save money in the long term. Logic would lead an observer to conclude that money would follow the evidence-based aspects of prevention, but it is of course not that simple. In the National Health Service, general practices are required to meet prevention targets, which are easier to achieve in the better-off areas where the prior probability of disease is obviously less. Payment is linked to the achievement of such targets.

In countries where patients subscribe to insurance plans, it is not at all unusual for such plans to concentrate on specialist and hospital services while completely ignoring primary care or preventive services. Some offer preventive services but require a co-payment, the patient having to pay some or all of the costs of the service. In more recent developments, insurance companies offer executive work-ups that include a large number of cardiac and life-style checks for those willing to pay. Some companies in Europe offer annual assessments as a condition of the continued membership of their schemes.

Medical inflation has outstripped annual inflation in most Western countries in recent years, and indeed nearly one third of bankruptcies in the USA have arisen because of medical bills. Those interested in prevention have, however, failed to persuade governments and insurers to transfer funds from curative medicine to prevention.

Health promotion

Health promotion is the enhancement of health at the physical, psychological, environmental and spiritual levels. Medicine has an input to physical and psychological parameters, and increasingly in terms of the environment, while also acknowledging the spiritual dimension of health.

It acts by protecting and improving health through behavioural, biological, socio-economic and environmental changes, involving, among others, politicians, environmentalists and public health and personal physicians. Action on tobacco-smoking is a good example of health promotion. Behaviour modification can occur through taxation at population level and through nicotine replacement at an individual level. Environmental change can help by prohibiting smoking indoors.

Health education

Whereas health promotion involves action at the population level, health education involves action at an individual or small group level. It includes the provision of readily available information on healthier life-styles and how to make the best use of the health services, with the intention of enabling rational health choices and ensuring an awareness of the factors determining the health of the community. Safe drinking is an example of health promotion, but informing people about safe limits is an educational exercise that may occur in schools or with the individual during a consultation with the doctor.

Health protection

This is derived from the tradition of public health and includes legal, fiscal and political measures and regulations to prevent ill-health, for example seat belt laws, taxes on cigarettes and alcohol, and the fluoridation of water. Doctors have an important role in influencing the development of healthy public policy because they hold positions of influence at the local, regional and national level.

Information about health

The general practice consultation affords an opportunity to provide information about health and illness that is specifically tailored to the patient's circumstances, through hand-drawn diagrams, leaflets or the addresses of self-help groups, for example. Doctors and patients are also increasingly using the internet. Health information makes up 40% of American websites, and it is estimated that there are over 1 million websites devoted to health world wide. Patients may want to discuss information downloaded from the Internet, which is a good example of the patient taking responsibility for his or her own health and using the doctor as a specialist adviser.

Table 1	**Relationship of risk factors to health**
Risk	**Impact on health**
Socio-economic	Strong links between poverty and ill-health
Environmental	Pollution, asthma, eczema
Genetic/family	Cystic fibrosis, schizophrenia, heart disease, diabetes
Occupational	Deafness, eczema/dermatitis, stress
Life-style	Alcohol, drugs, sexually transmitted diseases, diet
Travel	Communicable diseases
Behavioural	Risk-taking: bicycle helmets, unprotected sex
Poor education	Poor health practices in both the developed and the underdeveloped world
Illness	Psychiatric illness predisposes to suicide. Hyperlipidaema predisposes to myocardial infarction and hypertension to strokes
Cultural	Tolerance of alcohol: 'boys will be boys'. Resistance to genetic screening in Catholic and Muslim countries

General principles

- People are living longer due to the interplay of diet, education and, probably, medicine.
- Primary prevention permits the patient to remain disease free.
- Secondary prevention involves the early detection of disease.
- Tertiary prevention aims to minimise the progression of disease.
- GPs see individual patients 3–4 times/year and are well placed to encourage prevention.
- Those committed to prevention have difficulty in persuading funders to transfer money from curative to preventative.
- Health information comprises 40% of websites in the USA.

Practical issues

Primary care is generally considered to be a key place for prevention. At the practical level, however, barriers exist that interfere with the delivery of disease prevention and health promotion.

Patient barriers

Education

Education is a powerful agent for change. Between 10% and 20% of people in Western societies have trouble with both reading and writing. This has a direct effect as well as depriving a subgroup of the benefit of written materials on health education. Language problems may be mistaken for educational deficits, particularly among ethnic minorities or refugees. There are also important gender differences, women having a greater responsibility than men for the family's health. Educational programmes on health geared towards women can have dramatic results in areas such as fertility and childcare (Fig. 1).

Work

Unemployment affects up to 10% of the eligible working population and is itself a barrier to a healthy life. Within the unemployment statistics lie a group of long-term unemployed people who are likely to be poorly educated and poorly skilled. This subgroup is particularly vulnerable to ill-health as a direct effect of poverty.

In the working population, many people have to work overtime in order to make ends meet and may have little time left for a healthy life-style. Work-related stress is now at epidemic proportions, often leading to ill-health and absenteeism.

Peer pressure

Peer pressure has both positive and negative effects. The decline in acceptability of smoking among the middle classes is an example of the former. The latter is exemplified by the increase in smoking and alcohol consumption seen particularly among young women, and also by the experimentation with drugs often observed in the teenage years.

Enjoyment

The use of tobacco and alcohol is a good example of activities that are enjoyed by a large number of people. It is an uphill task trying to persuade people to give up, or cut down, on enjoyable activities, even if this is for their own good.

Barriers among professionals

Primary care professionals are in a good position to prevent some illnesses. Doctors may, however, lack the interest and motivation to avail themselves of the opportunities presented to discuss prevention. Some doctors see health promotion as unnecessarily meddlesome in patients'

lives and argue that the evidence for prevention is lacking in many areas (Skrabanek et al 1998).

Time is probably the biggest barrier to prevention and health promotion in general practice. It has been argued that the consultation provides exceptional opportunities for doctors to engage in prevention and modify help-seeking behaviour (Stott and Davis 1979). The consultation length is, however, still less than 10 minutes in most general practices, leaving little time for anything other than dealing with the presenting complaint. But the opportunities, particularly for secondary prevention in general practice, are enormous, for example:

- a good control of blood sugar level in diabetes
- a reduction of risk factors after myocardial infarction
- using inhaled steroids in asthma.

Who should do it?

Health promotion is an activity that is geared towards populations and is capable of raising the awareness of particular aspects of health. In a health-care system that is working well, public health departments can identify local or regional deficiencies in health and alert both the media and the primary care teams to the need to intervene effectively. GPs often overrate the influence of the media because their experience is frequently in the area of dealing with media-driven health scares that frighten rather than inform patients.

Antenatal and parentcraft classes are seen as good opportunities to promote health and provide both information and networks for pregnant women and their children. Such a group are naturally interested in doing their best for their children. However, young mothers sometimes find the content of such classes to be too technical for their understanding. The GP consultation rate of young mothers, particularly with their first child, is high because of preventable problems such as upper respiratory tract illness related to a high level of smoking in the home, and feeding difficulties, usually caused by over-feeding. Many health-care systems now have health visitors or public health nurses specially trained to deal with the problems of new parents.

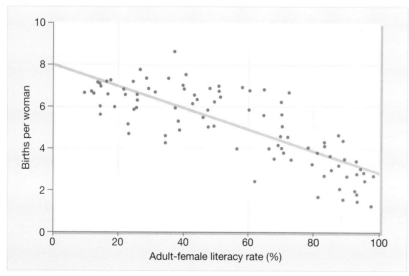

Fig. 1 **A little learning: fertility rate and female literacy 1990, births per woman.**

Examples of opportunities for prevention

Pre-conception

There is now good evidence that the administration of 0.8 mg folic acid in the 3 months prior to conception and during the first trimester significantly reduces the incidence of neural tube defects in the newborn. To get this message across, all the available opportunities have to be used at population and individual level: even the baker may help by fortifying bread with folic acid! A key obstacle, however, is that 30–40% of pregnancies are unplanned and women may not know that they are pregnant for 4–6 weeks, thereby missing out on the window of opportunity for preventing neural tube defects.

Respiratory infections and smokers

Because GPs see patients on average three times a year, they have an excellent opportunity to develop a good relationship with patients and also to use these consultations for prevention and the early detection of disease. A smoker presenting with signs of an upper or lower respiratory tract infection is, for example, likely to be more receptive to advice about smoking because of its demonstrable effects on the chest (the so-called 'teachable moment'). A respected doctor giving advice about smoking to someone with respiratory illness is thus in a good position to alter behaviour.

Alcohol and advice

Screening and brief intervention involves the routine or opportunistic screening of the general practice population to identify 'at-risk' drinkers (Box 1) and the subsequent delivery of brief structured advice (Box 2). This usually comprises 5–10 minutes of advice on reducing drinking, information on 'safe levels' of consumption (14 units per week for women and 21 for men) and brief counselling and/or referral.

The target population comprises those drinking at a hazardous (conferring the risk of harm) or harmful (causing harm) level. There is strong evidence that brief intervention is effective with excessive drinkers, reducing their consumption by 25–40% compared with that of controls receiving only assessment.

Box 1 The CAGE screening instrument

Two or more positive replies are suggestive of a problem drinker. Have you ever felt you:

1. should *cut* down on your drinking
2. get *annoyed* when your alcohol intake is discussed
3. ever felt *guilty* about your drinking
4. ever needed an *eye-opener* (early morning drink) to steady your nerves or get rid of a hangover.

Box 2 Brief intervention technique

1. Advise a reduction to a safe level
2. Outline the benefits of this reduction
3. Provide an information leaflet
4. Get the patient to monitor his or her progress with a diary
5. Follow up by consultation in person or by telephone
6. Suggest additional help such as counselling, Alcoholics Anonymous or disulfiram.

This takes 5–10 minutes

The age/sex register

Using the age/sex register, which is computerised in most practices, presents opportunities for health surveillance. One practice was, for example, concerned about the health of its growing population of over-75-year-old patients, particularly about the number living alone, about their daily support and about their hearing and vision. The practice therefore arranged to send a card on the patient's 75th birthday, signed by the patient's GP and enclosing a simple questionnaire addressing the concerns of the practice, together with a stamped addressed envelope. If the patient did not respond within 2 weeks, the health visitor was notified and a visit was arranged. The birthday card scheme was extremely popular with the over-75s, the questionnaire revealing them to be extremely robust and active, albeit a little hard of hearing.

How much advice?

This requires a surprising amount of judgement at the level of the individual patient. The degree of interest and motivation of the patient is important in prevention. Education has to be pitched both at a level and in a language that is understood by the patient, and information using visual and written material can be provided to individual patients by nurses and doctors. Patients are increasingly interested in website addresses (there being over a million health-oriented websites world wide) – see the bibliography list at the end of the book.

Whom to target?

The Family Heart Study involved women as well as men in its cardiovascular screening programme (Family Heart Study Group 1994); the women were seen to play an important role in modifying risk factors, especially in the area of nutrition and diet. There are also phases of life when people are interested in health matters, for example antenatally, as young parents and when recently retired. Children too can play an important part in bringing a health message to a parent who smokes, although the children of smokers are paradoxically more likely to smoke themselves. General practice is well suited to the support and monitoring tasks of secondary prevention.

Readiness to change behaviour

A model of behaviour for explaining readiness to change behaviour and habits now exists. The first phase is *pre-contemplation* in which the individual has not even begun to think about change. Another may be at the *contemplation* stage thinking about, for example, the effects of smoking on their health. The final stage is *ready to change*. This individual is worth identifying because the success rate is likely to be greatest.

Practical issues

- Lack of education and language problems are important barriers in prevention
- A familiar comfortable but unhealthy lifestyle is difficult to change.
- Shortage of time is a huge barrier to prevention in general practice.
- The media can frighten but finds it more difficult to inform patients.

Introduction and general overview

As with the rest of this book, this section is not intended to give a definitive, exhaustive account of all the causes of ill-health by age and sex, but good working knowledge of the main differences.

Consultation rates

In the UK and most other developed countries, day-to-day medical care is delivered through general practice. The on average just over three consultations per person on a GP's list per year conceals as Fig. 1 shows, quite big differences by age and sex. The highest consultation rates occur in the very young, in the elderly and in adult women generally. The lowest rates are in older and early teenage children of both sexes, and in younger men.

Common conditions

Overall, the most common conditions for which people consult a doctor are shown in Fig. 2. If the four respiratory diagnostic groups (upper respiratory tract infection, sore throat, asthma and lower respiratory tract infection) are aggregated, respiratory problems are by far the most prevalent causes of consultation. When the usual reasons for visiting the GP are analysed by age and sex, as in Table 1, there are, however, some interesting differences in pattern.

Young children mostly consult because of infections and allergies (asthma and eczema). By young adulthood, acne, drug abuse and accidents (trauma) have become common in males, and contraception and depression in females. In older adult males, backache, depression and anxiety are the most common problems, as in older females, although for them this is also the main reproductive phase (requiring antenatal care). High blood pressure (hypertension) starts to become a very common problem in both sexes in middle age, women also often being troubled by menopausal symptoms.

Thereafter, the chronic degenerative diseases of old age start to take over. In men, chronic obstructive airways disease, mostly what used to be known as 'chronic bronchitis', and caused largely by smoking and to a lesser extent other air pollutants, becomes common, as do various manifestations of heart disease. In women, osteoarthritis (joint disease from, in simple terms, 'wear and tear') commonly appears at an earlier age than it does in men and depression remains a common problem, but chronic lung and heart disease do not feature as prominently.

Prevention of ill-health

Of course, a great deal of activity in primary care is concerned not with treating illness but with trying to prevent it. As Table 1 shows, child health surveillance is one of the most frequent causes of consultation with children. This is associated with an extensive programme of immunisation against common infectious diseases. Serious infections, such as diphtheria and polio, which formerly killed and maimed thousands of children every year, have now been virtually wiped out in the developed world. Contraception is another major preventive activity, although the rate of therapeutic abortion (224 per 1000 live births in Scotland in 1998) still reflects a high rate of unwanted pregnancy.

Most developed countries have major screening programmes, particularly for the early detection of various forms of cancer. In the UK, the most important programmes cover the early detection of cervical and breast cancers in women. A most important feature of the UK system of general practice is that all individuals are registered with a GP. The population looked after by a general practice therefore consists mostly of people who are healthy and well, but they may still be contacted by health staff or use the practice for advice or other action to maintain their health and prevent illness.

In contrast, hospitals deal in a much more concentrated way with the serious end of the illness spectrum (Table 4).

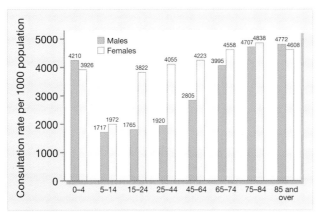

Fig. 1 **GP consultation rates per 1000 population by sex and age group: year ending December 1998.** Data from 40 general practices. (Data from Scottish Health Statistics 1999)

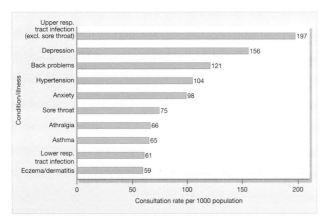

Fig. 2 **Top 10 consultation rates per 1000 population by condition/illness directing the consultations: year ending December 1998.** Data from 40 general practices, with complete data for the year ending December 1998. (Data from Scottish Health Statistics 1999)

Table 1 **The five most common reasons for consultation grouped by sex and age range (in order of frequency): year ending December 1998.** Data from 40 general practices. (From Scottish Health Statistics 1999)

	1	2	3	4	5
Males					
0–4	URTI (excl. sore throat)	Otitis media	CHS	Eczema/dermatitis	Diarrhoea ± vomiting
5–14	URTI (excl. sore throat)	Asthma	Sore throat	Otitis media	Eczema/dermatitis
15–24	Sore throat	Acne	Drug abuse	URTI (excl. sore throat)	Trauma – misc.
25–44	Back problems	Depression	Anxiety	URTI (excl. sore throat)	Trauma – misc.
45–64	Hypertension	Back problems	Depression	URTI (excl. sore throat)	Anxiety
65–74	Hypertension	URTI (excl. sore throat)	COAD	Coronary heart disease – misc.	Diabetes
75–84	Hypertension	COAD	URTI (excl. sore throat)	Heart failure	Coronary heart disease – misc
85 and over	URTI (excl. sore throat)	Heart failure	COAD	LRTI	Osteoarthritis
Females					
0–4	URTI (excl. sore throat)	CHS	Otitis media	Eczema/dermatitis	Diarrhoea ± vomiting
5–14	URTI (excl. sore throat)	Sore throat	Otitis media	Asthma	Eczema/dermatitis
15–24	Family planning – misc.	Oral contraceptive pill	Sore throat	Depression	URTI (excl. sore throat)
25–44	Depression	Anxiety	Antenatal	Back problems	URTI (excl. sore throat)
45–64	Menopause	Depression	Hypertension	Back problems	Anxiety
65–74	Hypertension	URTI (excl. sore throat)	Osteoarthritis	Depression	Back problems
75–84	Hypertension	URTI (excl. sore throat)	Osteoarthritis	Back problems	Depression
85 and over	URTI (excl. sore throat)	Heart failure	Trauma – misc.	Hypertension	Urinary tract infection

1 Data based on 40 General Practices with complete data for year ending December 1998.

Key to abbreviations used: ±: with or without. CHS: Child Health Surveillance. URTI: Upper respiratory tract infection. LRTI: Lower respiratory tract infection. COAD: Chronic obstructive airway disease.

Table 2 **Abdominal pain in general practice**

- Myocardial infarction may present as severe dyspepsia
- Intussusception
- Ectopic pregnancy
- Diabetic ketoacidosis
- Testicular torsion
- Appendicitis
- Gastroenteritis

Table 3 **Non-emergency abdominal pain in general practice**

- Dyspepsia (48%)
- Irritable bowel syndrome (23%)
- Psychological causes (15%)
- Mittelschmerz (4%)
- Carcinoma of the stomach or rectum
- Crohn's disease and ulcerative colitis
- Pelvic inflammatory disease

Table 4 **The 10 most common reasons for hospital admission in Scotland, 1998/1999**

- Digestive system (14%)
- Malignant neoplasms (cancers) (10.9%)
- Injury, poisonings etc. (8.7%)
- Heart disease (7.7%)
- Respiratory system (6.8%)
- Musculoskeletal system (4.9%)
- Urinary system (3.4%)
- Skin diseases (3.2%)
- Other circulatory diseases (not heart disease) (2.9%)
- Eye diseases (2.6%)

(Data from Scottish Health Statistics 1999)

Example: acute abdominal pain

The example of acute abdominal pain is included here as a specific illustration of the relationship between general practice and specialist (hospital) care. It also illustrates another important feature of the work of a generalist. He or she has to be able to distinguish (often quickly and in an emergency) the need for urgent admission for surgical or other emergency treatment in a situation where both minor and serious causes of disease may present with very similar initial symptoms. Patients consult frequently with abdominal pain, yet only a minority are referred to hospital.

Children

Between 10% and 20% of children suffer from recurrent abdominal pain, defined as 'more than 3 attacks within 3 months sufficient to disrupt activity'. (Apley 1975). Parents will worry that such pains are caused by 'grumbling appendicitis', among many other things. Diseases of the urinary tract account for some of the organic causes of recurrent abdominal pain, but other physical causes are extremely rare.

There is a strong psychological element to abdominal pain in children. A good history exploring the parent–child relationship, attitudes to food, sleep and school, and teasing and bullying, together with an examination of the abdomen, will reassure most patients. A mid-stream urine sample is probably the most valuable investigation, and advice about diet will resolve most cases of constipation. The avoidance of over-investigation is an important aspect of management of recurrent abdominal pain in children.

Adults

Abdominal pain in adults can present to the GP as either an emergency or a non-emergency. The acute abdomen in general practice includes a wide range of conditions (Table 2). All these conditions are rare, with a dramatic fall-off in the incidence of appendicitis in recent years.

Non-emergency abdominal pain

This is much more common in general practice than is the acute abdomen (Table 3). Most cases of an acute abdomen need urgent referral to hospital, whereas non-emergency abdominal pain can mostly be diagnosed and treated within general practice with occasional investigation and/or referral for a specialist opinion.

Introduction and general overview

- This section outlines how patterns of ill-health and acute illness differ in males and females, and at different ages in life.
- Patterns of illness presented to GPs are contrasted with those encountered in hospital practice.
- Abdominal pain is used as an example to illustrate the relationship between general and specialist practice.

Children

Age profile (0–12 years)

In the space of little more than a decade, a helpless baby weighing about 7 pounds develops into a mini-person of about 7 stone, with complex language and social skills, intricate motor skills and an astonishing range of general knowledge. This period of development is concerned primarily with physical, social, intellectual and emotional growth (Table 1).

Table 1 **Infant development**

2–3 months	Sits with good head control
4–6 months	Attempts self-feeding
5–6 months	Sits without support
6 months onwards	Recognisable speech development
7–8 months	Stands holding onto furniture, etc.
9–12 months	Drinks from a cup
12–14 months	Walks well
16–18 months	Kicks a ball

The main stresses of childhood are related to the early need for dependence on adults and the later need to reduce that dependence in order to develop as a fully independent person (Box 1). Early emotional bonding (initially with a single adult, who may not necessarily be the natural mother) is essential for normal emotional development. Although children are resilient, serious emotional damage leading to antisocial behaviour and delinquency can result from insecure child–parent relationships.

Changing social structures with, in many developed countries, a breakdown of traditional stable families, an increased number of changes of partner and a rising divorce rate, increased lone parenting (Box 2) and fewer prospects of stable employment may make it more difficult to create safe and stable conditions for child development.

Main acute health problems

Given good nutrition and a safe and healthy environment, childhood should be one of life's healthiest periods. An unfortunate minority of children suffer from chronic ailments, the most common chronic ailments in childhood – asthma and eczema of the skin – both being associated with allergy. On the other hand, all children contract frequent minor illnesses as they come into contact for the first

Box 1 **Main stages of socio-emotional development.** (After Erikson 1968)

- *Birth – 18 months: trust versus mistrust.* Children learn to trust, or mistrust, that their needs will be met by the world, especially by their mother.
- *18 months to 3 years: autonomy versus shame, doubt.* Children learn to exercise will, to make choices and to control themselves, or they become uncertain and doubt that they can do things by themselves.
- *3–6 years: initiative versus guilt.* Children learn to initiate activities and enjoy their accomplishments, acquiring direction and purpose. If they are not allowed initiative, they feel guilty for their attempts at independence.
- *6–12 years: industry versus inferiority.* Children develop a sense of industry and curiosity and are eager to learn, or they feel inferior and lose interest in the tasks before them.
- *Adult: identity versus role confusion.* Adolescents come to see themselves as unique and integrated persons with an ideology, or else they become confused about what they want out of life.

Box 2 **UK divorce rates**

In the UK, divorce has increased by over 600% over the past 20 years. One in three marriages is now likely to end in divorce, 60% involving children under 16 years of age. Each year, approximately 160 000 children see their parents separate, and the proportion of lone-parent families has increased, from 8% in 1971 to 14% in 1987 (OPCS 1988).

time with one or other of the several hundred different acute viral infections that may affect them. These generally cause minor and self-limiting acute respiratory and/or gastrointestinal symptoms. Although one must still be alert, particularly for meningitis (see Appendix 5, p. 103), the serious

infections of children are largely eliminated by immunisation. Through a combination of inexperience and an urge to explore and experiment, accidents are the most common serious threat to health in childhood.

Acute self-limiting infections

These are by far the most common cause of illness in childhood. The way in which illness presents varies to some extent with the age of the child. There is usually a prodromal stage during which the child is obviously 'not himself', i.e. not as active as usual and/or not eating well, perhaps obviously hot and sweaty or known to be pyrexial because the parents have taken the child's body temperature. The main features of the presentation are therefore symptoms of general malaise with pyrexia.

Specific symptoms (e.g. cough, sore throat or diarrhoea) may help to localise the main site of the infection, but many viruses have multi-system effects. Up until the age of about 4 or 5 years, children may not identify specific features (e.g. sore throat and earache) well themselves. It is, however, important to identify the site of infection. Throat and ear infections and short-lived attacks of gastroenteritis are extremely common and generally innocuous. Serious infections such as pneumonia and meningitis can, however, present with the same general features of malaise and pyrexia. It is therefore important to be confident of the diagnosis otherwise the child should be regarded as having a *'pyrexia of uncertain origin'* and observed and/or investigated accordingly.

A case study

On pages 18–21, there are some general points about clinical problem-solving, the case below illustrating some particular points about dealing with young children.

Mrs Ingram brings her 3-month-old son, Darren, to you because he has 'just not been himself'. He is bottle-fed but has not been finishing his feeds. He is irritable and crying much more than usual, but in between bouts of crying he is quite alert, playful and attentive. He started off with a cold a few days ago. According to his mother, 'his nose is all bunged up and his breathing is heavy'. She has also noticed that Darren is very sweaty and hot to touch. He does not have any skin rash.

Case history

On examination you find that Darren's right eardrum is distended and acutely inflamed (Fig. 1). This is the typical appearance of acute otitis media.

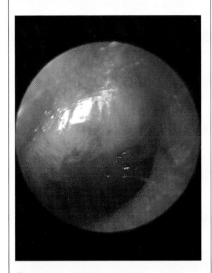

Fig. 1 **The tympanic membrane in acute otitis media.** Source: Stafford and Youngs (1999).

Unfortunately, small children cannot tell us what they feel to be wrong with them: even once they are able to speak, they cannot localise the site of a pain very accurately until they are approaching school age. Being off feeds, crying and irritability are non-specific behavioural changes that simply tell us that the child is unwell. The degree of these general changes is, however, a guide to the seriousness of the illness: extreme irritability, a complete disinterest in play, drowsiness and a lack of alertness are, for example, indications of possibly life-threatening illness (e.g. septicaemia or meningitis – see Appendix 5, p. 103).

Judging by these general symptoms, Darren does not seem to be seriously ill at the moment (although the situation may change rapidly in young children). We know that infections are the most common causes of acute illness at this age. This is also suggested by his being sweaty and hot to touch, and a raised body temperature will confirm the likelihood of infection.

The infection could theoretically, be anywhere – urinary system, gastrointestinal system, etc. – but there are a number of reasons why it is highly likely to be in the upper respiratory tract:

- Upper respiratory infections are known to be by far the most usual kind of infection at this age.
- Darren has recently had the symptoms of a common cold.
- We know that, once mucosal resistance to infection has been reduced by viral inflammation, such as occurs with a 'cold', other 'secondary' bacterial infections may follow. These secondary infections tend to occur in parts adjacent to the upper respiratory tract, most commonly the ears and the lower respiratory tract.

Conclusion

Some examples of serious threats to the health of children are given in Table 2, but it is equally important to try to avoid illness by promoting the sort of healthy action shown in Table 3. Some common accidental injuries and examples of preventive measures are given in Appendix 6, p. 103.

Table 2 **Emergencies and rarities to be alert for**

- Dehydration
- Accidents
- Non-accidental injury
- Respiratory distress
  - severe asthma
  - laryngotracheobronchitis (croup)
  - bronchiolitis
  - foreign bodies
- Overwhelming infections (e.g. meningitis)
- Surgical emergencies (e.g. intussusception or torsion of the testes)

Table 3 **Main targets for prevention and health promotion**

- The promotion of breast-feeding
- The avoidance of secondary smoking
- Healthy life-styles – nutrition, exercise, anti-smoking, anti-drugs
- Early socialisation – playgroups and nurseries
- Healthy parenting
- Immunisation
- Accident prevention – homes, schools, road safety
- Beware of strangers

Box 3 **Communicating with younger children**

The child patient should always be treated as important in his or her own right, so it is important to talk to, and pay attention to, the child directly, not just through the parent. You need to talk quietly and move slowly so as not to startle the child and explain what you are going to do, even if the child may not seem old enough to understand completely. Watching the behaviour of the child can be very informative and it is useful to have some toys (but not soft toys, which transmit infections) in the surgery, not just to keep children amused but to watch how interested they are in play. It is usually best to watch the child unobtrusively to begin with, without appearing to pay too much attention to him or her, until the child starts to show interest in you. It is usually best to get down to the child's eye level by kneeling crouching or sitting on the floor. With an older child you can start by talking about toys or television programmes. Some children seem hell bent on destroying the surgery but it is usually best not to restrain them unless they are putting themselves in danger and to discourage parents from over-reacting, which seems to make bad behaviour worse. Paying some direct attention to the child usually helps. It should be possible to examine most older children without too much difficulty but younger children may need to be gently restrained by the parent whilst you examine ears and throat.

Children

- Paradoxically, good upbringing of children requires that they initially have a secure, highly dependent relationship with parents, but that parents subsequently allow the child to develop his or her independence of them.

- Infections are the commonest cause of illness in childhood and are mostly self-limiting. The most important signs of serious illness are often behavioural effects – irritability, disinterest in play and drowsiness or lack of alertness.

- Domestic accidents are a major preventable cause of illness.

- Despite the fact that much illness is prevented by immunisation there is still much scope for further preventive action in e.g. promotion of breast feeding, accident prevention and avoidance of secondary smoking.

Adults

Age group profile (approximately 20–45 years)

During this period of the family life cycle (see p. 26), the young adult usually uproots from the original family and establishes an independent existence, perhaps in turn setting up a new family unit (although this traditional family unit pattern is now less common; see p. 28). This period of life is therefore mostly preoccupied with career development, child-rearing and an attempt to achieve financial and domestic security. Maslow's hierarchy (Fig. 1) is a useful model for understanding what motivates people's behaviour, particularly during this stage of achievement in life.

Although the relationship between motivation and stress is complex, current trends in competitive modern life are likely to be an increasing cause of conflict, particularly in terms of high unemployment, insecurity and an increased workload for those who remain in work, coupled with decreased social security and increasing economic pressure. It is a particularly important period during which to establish healthy life-style patterns, which will pay dividends much later in life. By the early 40s or even earlier, there is already some premature mortality and morbidity, mainly in men as a result of the so-called 'diseases of life-style', particularly ischaemic heart disease.

Main acute health problems

This is a relatively healthy period for men, during which their GP consultation rate is particularly low. Women experience a much higher prevalence of health problems during this period, much of it related to reproduction and child-rearing. Many regard this difference in health between men and women as being yet another expression of social inequality arising from gender bias. The particular health problems of men and women are dealt with on pages 46–51. Apart from these, accidents and mental health problems (including marital and other relationship difficulties, e.g. at work, and addiction to alcohol and drugs) tend to typify this period in both sexes. Although women experience higher morbidity during this period, their overall death rate is approximately half that of men, primarily because men are much more likely to die from accidents, violence and suicide.

Acute infections

The most common problems are still acute infections, mostly minor and self-limiting, and predominantly of the upper respiratory tract.

Respiratory tract infections

Most of these are caused by viral infection, but the combination of fever, tonsillar exudate and anterior cervical lymphadenopathy has been found to raise the probability of streptococcal isolation to 42% (from 3% in patients with none of these findings), identifying those who are most likely to benefit from antibiotic treatment (phenoxymethylpenicillin, or erythromycin for those who are penicillin sensitive). *Haemophilus influenzae*, *Chlamydia* and *Mycoplasma* are occasional causative agents, particularly when the cough is troublesome and the symptoms are prolonged. These pathogens are resistant to penicillin, so other newer antibiotics may be required.

Urinary tract infections   Urinary tract infections (pp 78–79) are quite common in women but not in men (for anatomical and other reasons). There is an increasing awareness of the need to detect and prevent the progression of underlying renal disease, although this is relatively rare. There should consequently be a greater readiness to investigate the renal tract, particularly when there are possible 'risk factors' such as urinary infections in childhood and relapsing or persistent infections with the same organism.

Gastrointestinal infections (see also pp 52–53 and pp 84–85) Gastrointestinal infection may, for reasons that are not entirely clear, be increasing in prevalence, and the average adult can expect to have several episodes of diarrhoea and/or vomiting per year. Most are short lived and should be self-treated. Only about a third of cases have an identifiable infectious cause, *Salmonellae*, *Shigellae* and *Campylobacter* being among the most important organisms. In general, however, antibiotic and other specific therapy is unhelpful in most of these cases. Investigation is therefore usually confined to those with particularly severe illness or where there is a risk to public health (e.g. food-handlers and health-care workers). Chronic infection of the bowel by *Helicobacter pylori* (see p. 82) has recently been recognised to be the most important cause of peptic ulcer and other gastrointestinal diseases.

Injuries

Injuries, particularly to the muscles (rather than bones or joints) are also common, *acute low back pain* perhaps epitomising this group of complaints. It has been estimated that 9 out of 10 people have at least one episode of acute low back pain in their lifetime, and it is a leading cause of sickness absence. In most cases, no precise

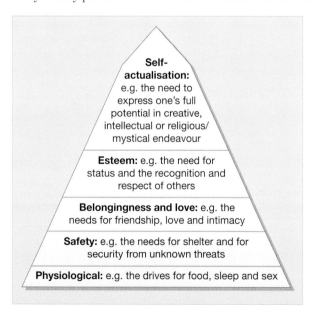

Fig. 1   **Maslow's hierarchy of needs.** Adapted from Maslow (1954).

anatomical diagnosis can be made. About 1 in 10 patients also have sciatica, indicating the irritation or compression of a lumbosacral nerve root. Overall, more than 80% of sufferers recover within a month, and further investigation (generally computed tomography or magnetic resonance imaging, and/or myelography – plain X-rays being of little or no diagnostic value) should be reserved for those in whom severe symptoms persist for more than about 2 months. Approximately 1% of sufferers will come to require surgical treatment (see p. 77).

Minor psychological disorders

These are particularly common in this age group (see the case study below and pp 64–69).

A case study

Case history

Roger Chalmers is a 35-year-old accountant. His wife works as a schoolteacher, and they have three children aged between 2 and 9 years. Roger has recently been feeling 'tired all the time' despite going to bed reasonably early. He tends to wake up during the early morning and has difficulty getting back to sleep. He has also had a lot of headaches recently, as well as other aches and pains. In particular, he has had some pains in his chest which he is especially worried about: his father died from a heart attack when he was aged about 75. Roger is trying to build up a new accountancy firm with another new partner, and it has been a bit of a struggle. They both work very long hours, take a lot of work home and rarely go on holiday. Roger and his wife are not getting on very well, either: they tend to snap at each other all the time and get very little time to themselves.

Comments

- The most important point here is that diagnosis of psychological conditions should not be made by default, i.e. by 'excluding the physical', but by making the psychological diagnosis on positive grounds. There are, for example, several positive indicators of a psychological diagnosis here – the presence of obvious stress, the disturbance of sleep pattern, the unexplained lassitude and irritability.
- On the other hand, there are no positive indicators of any important

physical diagnosis, so why look for it? The complaint of chest pain might sound worrying, but it is much more likely to have a psychological foundation. The probability of any serious pathology is extremely low and can be virtually eliminated by a few well-chosen questions.

- Roger's personal complaints cannot satisfactorily be dealt in isolation from a consideration of his work and family as he needs to find a better balance between work and leisure. It might help to arrange some joint sessions with his wife, if she is willing to attend, and/or to arrange some more specialised counselling.

- This is an age at which many men become worried (usually unnecessarily) about heart attacks. The opportunity may be taken to educate them about the actual risks (which are probably much less than they fear) and the really useful steps (principally not smoking cigarettes) that they can take to minimise the risks. There is a small group of individuals who have a very strong hereditary risk; this is suggested by the death of a father or brothers at a young age, for example under 60 years (and not 75 as in the case of Roger's father). These high-risk individuals may need further investigation for individual risk factors (e.g. blood lipid levels).

Conclusion

Some examples (although not a comprehensive list) of serious threats to health in adults are given in Table 1, but it is equally important to try to avoid illness by promoting the sorts of healthy actions shown in Table 2.

Table 1 Emergencies and rarities to be alert for

- Respiratory obstruction/failure
  - severe acute asthma/anaphylaxis
  - foreign bodies
- Circulatory collapse
  - acute myocardial infarction
  - pulmonary embolism
- Internal bleeding
  - intracranial
  - intestinal
  - ruptured aortic aneurysm

Table 2 Main targets for prevention and health promotion

- Healthy life-style – nutrition, smoking, alcohol, drugs, skin care
- Accident prevention
- Safe sex
- Immunisation and foreign travel
- Early diagnosis and screening
  - cervical and breast cancer
  - testicular and prostatic cancer
  - bowel cancer
  - ischaemic heart disease risk factors
  - skin cancer
  - hypertension
  - renal disease
  - diabetes
  - glaucoma

Box 1 Main measures of obesity

Body Mass Index (BMI)
The BMI is the main measure of obesity:

$$BMI = weight (kg)/height (m^2)$$
E.g. a person of 1.8 m height and 70 kg weight has a BMI of:

$$70/1.8 \times 1.8 = 70/3.24 = 21.6$$

A BMI of 25.0–29.9 is taken to indicate overweight
A BMI over 30 indicates obesity

Waist circumference
Waist circumference is a better measurement of intra-abdominal fat which also highly predicts health risk. Risk of cardiovascular disease in particular is increased if waist circumference exceeds 94 cm (37 inches) for men and 80 cm (32 inches) for women

Inspired by BMJ special edition 5 October 2002

Adults

- Early adulthood is mostly pre-occupied with establishing an independent existence – career development, child rearing and achieving financial and domestic security.
- Women present more problems than men to health

care, largely due to reproduction and child rearing, but men may avoid seeking help and are more likely to die from accidents, violence and suicide.

- The main problems – infections, injuries and psychological problems – are

mainly dealt with wholly within general practice.

- In later adulthood one of the main tasks is to prevent avoidable early deaths e.g. from heart attacks and cancer.

The elderly I

Table 1 **Some effects of growing old**

	Effect	Possible cause(s)
Skin	The skin loses elasticity, becoming thinner, drier and less flexible ('wrinkly')	Long-term exposure to sunlight (ultraviolet radiation), the effects being greater in, for example, white-skinned people living in hot countries
Body fat	Often increases, although the overall weight may not increase because there may be an associated decrease in muscle mass and bone density. Fat deposits around the waist (an 'apple' as opposed to 'pear' shape) are associated with increased cardiovascular risk	Generally poor nutrition and over-eating rather than ageing *per se*
Hearing	Most people develop high-tone deafness, even from the age of about 40 onwards. By the mid-60s, many people have difficulty following a conversation, especially if there is much background noise	At least some of this hearing loss is caused by damage from high noise levels, e.g. loud music and industrial machinery. The use of ear protection helps to preserve good hearing
Eyesight	The lens of the eye loses flexibility, rather like the skin, so cannot expand and contract as readily. This causes difficulty in focussing down on small print (presbyopia or 'long-sightedness'), starting in most people by about age 50 or earlier. Brighter light is needed to see as well as before, and colour vision, depth perception and night vision are all diminished. Cataracts (permanent clouding of the lenses, obscuring vision) may occur	Smoking, exposure to radiation (including ultraviolet) and other oxidation effects may be factors in the development of cataract in particular
Musculoskeletal system	The muscles and tendons become weaker and more prone to injury, and the bones lose their density. Both effects, particularly the loss of bone density, are greater in women than men	Both effects result largely from a change in the balance between the building-up and breaking-down of the tissues. Gradually with age, more tissue is being broken down than replaced. Regular exercise may retard this process
Brain and nervous system	Although there is a considerable loss of brain tissue with age, this does not necessarily cause intellectual deterioration as there are various compensatory mechanisms	Alzheimer's disease and cerebrovascular disease are the main causes of dementia. Simple forgetfulness is, however, almost universal even in younger people and is *not* a sign of impending dementia
Other body systems	The lungs and gastrointestinal system are less affected by ageing than are the cardiovascular and renal system	Cardiovascular deterioration can be reduced by improving risk factors such as smoking, overweight and salt and fat intake. There is also a significant hereditary element

causing deafness, exposure to ultraviolet radiation, toxic chemicals in the environment and so on.

By middle age, a high percentage of people have developed high blood pressure, coronary artery disease, diabetes, osteoarthritis, chronic bronchitis and other so-called 'degenerative' diseases (Table 2). Although these diseases can kill, and a small proportion of middle-aged people die prematurely from myocardial infarction (a 'heart attack' or 'coronary') in particular, most of these diseases follow a chronic, long-term course, often with increasing disability. Cancers, especially of the bowel and lung, and of the breast in women, are a major cause of premature death, although not by any means inevitably, as treatment, particularly when applied at an early stage, becomes increasingly effective.

The 'demographic time bomb'

The population profiles of developed and under-developed countries are very different (Fig. 1) because, in underdeveloped countries, many more people die prematurely, particularly in childhood, as was the case in developed countries 50 or 100 years ago. In the 1850s, an American could expect to live to about 39 years; by 1950 this had risen to 55, and in the 21st century the average American will live well into his 70s.

The increased in survival in developed countries has been caused mainly by improvements in public health (clean water and hygiene,

Old age is the final phase in the family life cycle (see p. 26). Most people spend about half of their lives in this later stage of children having grown up and 'fled the nest', living alone together as a couple again, to be followed later by retirement and eventually death.

It is not until middle age that most people start to experience the effects of growing old (Table 1). However, not all of these are strictly caused by ageing; most in fact result from the exposure of the body over time to various damaging influences such as smoking, alcohol, over-eating and poor nutrition, a lack of exercise, excessive noise levels

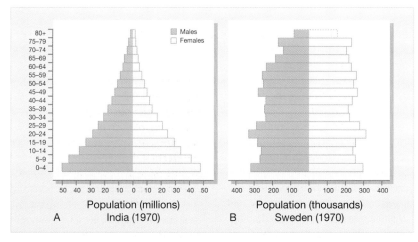

Fig. 1 **Age structure of populations: (a)** India, **(b)** Sweden.

Table 2 Common 'degenerative' diseases of middle age and the elderly

Body system	Diseases	Brief description
The heart and circulatory system	High blood pressure, coronary heart disease and stroke	These are the general effects of 'hardening of the arteries' (arteriosclerosis), in which the main blood vessels of the body lose their flexibility and become narrower. Having high blood pressure increases the risk of coronary heart disease and strokes. Coronary heart disease is the usual cause of a 'heart attack', in which the patient has severe chest pain. With a stroke, the patient usually develops a sudden paralysis of one side of the body, often with some loss of ability to speak
All systems	Cancers	Cancer may affect any part of the body, the most common sites being the large bowel, lungs and skin, the breasts and reproductive organs in women, and the prostate in men
The lungs	Chronic bronchitis	Chronic bronchitis (like lung cancer) is a disease that usually results from smoking. It causes chronic shortness of breath, coughing and wheezing, which can ultimately be severely disabling
The joints	Osteoarthritis	Although there are other causes of arthritis, osteoarthritis is the most common. Very many older people are affected, albeit to a greater or lesser effect, because it is thought to be an almost universal condition caused primarily by 'wear and tear' on the joints
The brain	Dementia	About a fifth of those over 80 are demented, that is, they have a severe deterioration in mental function to the extent that they usually cannot look after themselves. Dementia is mainly the result of a largely unknown process called Alzheimer's disease and is permanent, but there are some causes of reversible confusion in the elderly that may have to be differentiated (see Box 1, p. 44)

Box 1 Recent advances

- Chronic inflammation has a key role in the abnormal processes related to aging, including changes in body composition, congestive heart failure and possibly dementia. Anti-inflammatory drugs such as aspirin and non-steroidal anti-inflammatory drugs (NSAIDs, e.g. ibuprofen) may protect against cardiovascular disease, dementia and cancer but at the moment their general use is prohibited by adverse effects (such as gastrointestinal bleeding).
- Increased oxidative stress is a key aspect of aging. Vitamins E and C and the trace element Selenium may give some protection against oxidative stress but these effects are not yet definitely proven.
- Control of high systolic blood pressure is important in preventing stroke.
- Targeted and coordinated home health care has been provided to improve the health of older people with chronic disease and to reduce admissions to hospital. Exercise programmes can increase walking capacity and ability to look after oneself.

Adapted from: Pahor and Applegate (1997)

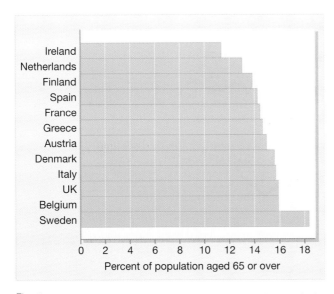

Fig. 2 **Percentage of the population aged over 65 (EU countries).**

improved housing and nutrition) rather than by medical treatment. Whereas a 50-year-old might have been considered 'old' in the 19th century, in the 20th and early 21st centuries 'old' is generally considered to be over 75. In Britain in the early 1900s, 12% of deaths occurred in the first year of life and 65% of people had died before reaching 65 years old, the corresponding figures today are 1% and 19% (Fig. 2).

Older people are also increasingly healthy, and there is an increasing emphasis on preserving health and fitness into old age by living healthier life-styles and aggressively identifying and treating disorders, for example hypertension and diabetes, that lead to disabling consequences such as stroke and heart failure (see Box 1). Many feel, however, that this will not greatly reduce the eventual need for health care, merely postponing it. Provided

that they can make adequate financial provision for 20 or more years of retirement, and provided that they have adequate social, health and welfare support, most of our current elderly population will continue to lead a fulfilling existence, many turning to new pastimes and new family roles, for example as grandparents. Fewer than 5% of those over 65 years old are in residential or nursing homes, and even at over 85, 80% still live in their own homes.

Although older people have poorer health than younger people, ageing does not cause disease: older people with better health habits live healthier for longer. Regular physical activity can 'rejuvenate' physical capacity by 10–15 years.

The elderly II

What is ageing?

Biological ageing

Table 1 (p. 42) shows some of the biological effects of ageing. These mostly result in a reduction in physical prowess and stamina. The effects on eyesight and hearing are particularly important as they can affect the ability to function from day to day and interfere with social processes.

Psychological ageing

It is generally thought that people can 'keep themselves young' by thinking positively and continuing to be engaged in useful and interesting tasks or hobbies, physical activities and sports, and by keeping up their social network. Up to a quarter of people aged over 65, rather more of those in residential care, are, however, estimated to suffer from depressive illness, and the incidence of suicide rises in the elderly, particularly in men. Depression, once identified, usually responds well to drug therapy, and the effects are therefore largely preventable. Severe depressive illness may be mistaken for dementia (which is on the whole not treatable) and therefore has to be carefully differentiated from it (Boxes 1 and 2).

Social ageing

Middle to old age can be a time of great social change, most of which may be interpreted as loss. People, for example, retire and may see themselves as no longer productive. Income drops, often drastically. Children leave home, and there are changes in role and social status. Many people move to a smaller house and may lose their neighbourhood friends and networks in the process, these social networks needing to be re-formed. Friends, relatives and spouses become seriously ill and die, and loneliness can set in (Box 3). Some elderly eventually become incapable of independent existence and need to move into residential care.

All of these effects are potentially depressing, but many people can maintain a positive attitude. Flexibility is thought to be the key here: those who age successfully are usually good at establishing new friends, maintaining family and social networks, developing new interests, managing their finances for retirement and continuing to fulfil a useful role in society through volunteer work or new family roles, such as being closely involved with their grandchildren (Box 4).

These effects are interactive but have been artificially separated here to illustrate the issues involved. It may, for example, be possible to ameliorate some of the biological effects of ageing by taking positive psychological and social action.

Box 1 Some potentially reversible causes of apparent dementia or confusional state in the elderly

True dementia is permanent and incurable. It is therefore particularly important not to miss potentially treatable causes of similar symptoms:

- prescription drugs
- alcohol and illicit drugs
- carbon monoxide
- heavy metal (e.g. lead) poisoning
- metabolic disorder, e.g. hypothyroidism
- encephalopathy, e.g. kidney or liver failure
- poor nutrition, e.g. folate or thiamine deficiency
- an intracranial lesion, e.g. a tumour or chronic subdural haematoma
- various vascular causes, e.g. atherosclerosis and embolic disease
- depressive illness
- acute infections, particularly of the lungs and urinary tract.

Box 2 Abbreviated mental test score

This is a simple test of intellectual capacity. A low score indicates possible intellectual impairment, although further detailed examination and testing would be required to confirm this and to elucidate the cause.
   Ask the patient:

1. Their age
2. The time (to the nearest hour)
3. Address – e.g. 42 West Street – for recall at end of test: this should be repeated by the patient to ensure that it has been heard correctly
4. Current year
5. Name of hospital (or place the patient is being seen)
6. Recognition of two people
7. Date of birth
8. Years of the First World War
9. Name of the present monarch
10. Count backwards from 20 to 1

Source: Hodkinson (1972). Quoted by Wattis J 1996 Caring for older people: what an old age psychiatrist does. BMJ 313: 101–104.

Box 3 Loneliness in the elderly

One in three elderly people feels lonely. There is a serious problem in about 10%, those most likely to be affected being very old people, widows and widowers, and people affected by disability. Lonely people who are reluctant to go out may be troubled by depression, agarophobia (a fear of open spaces), deafness or urinary incontinence, all of which may respond to treatment.
   Possible signs of loneliness are:

- verbal outpouring
- a prolonged holding of one's arm or hand
- body language with a defeated demeanour and tightly crossed arms and legs
- drab clothing.

Adapted from Forbes (1996)

Case studies

Case history

Middle age – hormone replacement therapy

The doctor was called to a house by the police because one of his patients, Mrs X, aged about 48, had attempted to stab her husband with a kitchen knife. The outcome of this was that she had been suffering from increasing irritability, very frequent 'hot flushes' and other signs of severe menopausal syndrome for several months. Her husband was a violent alcoholic, and on this particular night everything suddenly 'snapped'. This might well have happened anyway, but the menopausal symptoms seem to have reduced Mrs X to breaking point.

Once she was established on hormonal replacement therapy, she felt much better and much more able to take control of her life. In the end, she left her husband and established herself on her own very happily. The last time the doctor saw her, she said that there was 'no looking back' and that it was the best thing she had ever done for herself. No police action was taken over the attempted stabbing.

Case history

Middle age – heart disease

Mr K is a baker aged 60. He attended in a state of some shock because his brother, who was some 6 years younger than him, had just died suddenly from a heart attack, and the event had suddenly made Mr K think about his own health and mortality. He was in fact at an increased risk of having a heart attack himself for a number of reasons. There was a strong history of heart disease in the males in his family, he smoked and was overweight, and his blood cholesterol level was found to be high. The unfortunate death of his brother gave us an opportunity at least to take preventive action with Mr K.

It is not at all uncommon for men to avoid contact with the medical services for most of their lives, only to consult too late when an acute event acts as a precipitant. It is interesting that once Mr K was more comfortable with medical contact, he revealed some other problems, for example that he had been suffering from sexual impotence for a number of years (probably related to his circulatory difficulties) and that this had caused some problems within his marriage. The impotence was relatively easy to treat, which much improved his quality of life.

Case history

Elderly – confusional state

Mrs B is an 85-year-old living on her own. Her daughter had contacted the health visitor to say that the house was dirty and smelly, that Mrs B was not looking after herself and that she was 'getting senile'. The daughter and her husband seemed to be applying pressure for Mrs B to go into a home. Until recently, however, Mrs B had been doing all her own shopping every day and looking after herself in all respects. The situation was brought to a head when the daughter found Mrs B in bed, obviously confused – not knowing who her daughter was – and incontinent of both urine and faeces.

Although this sounds to be a seriously demented state, the old lady in fact proved to have a severe urinary tract infection, diabetes and cataracts (a condition seriously affecting her eyesight). Once these conditions had been satisfactorily treated, her apparent 'dementia' (in fact, a reversible confusional state; see Box 1) disappeared and she was once again able to live on her own.

Box 4   Standards for residential homes for the elderly

- personal choice in food, clothing, form of address, social activities, daily routine, general practitioner
- privacy
- an easily accessible complaints procedure
- an advocacy system for residents
- personal control of finance and medication where possible
- access to a full range of diversional activities
- access to community, health and social services
- an individualized care plan

Source: British Geriatrics Society. Policy statement No. 4: private and voluntary homes. London: British Geriatric Society, 1990. Cited by: Wanklyn P 1996.

Box 5

Former Prime Minister James Callaghan, interviewed in the *Independent on Sunday* after the publication of a new biography by Kenneth Morgan, reflects at the age of 85 on what remains: he reads a lot, including a poem each day; he writes occasional articles; keeps in touch with his large family; and helps with the washing up 'sometimes'. As the interviewer leaves, he is shown a photograph of the 1979 Cabinet: 'the smiling faces … turned into a roll call of death. "Gone, gone, gone … It's extraordinary," he concluded sadly. 'All that lot have gone …."'

As quoted by Currie C 1997. Old fools, rogues, lovers, and sages. BMJ, 315: 1102.

The elderly

- Improved public health and environmental measure are the main reasons why people live increasingly longer in developed countries.
- Nevertheless people continue to die prematurely from preventable causes.
- Today, most people should be able to lead a healthy life well into their seventies.
- Most of this depends more on social, economic and life-style measures than on medical intervention, but medicine particularly helps those individuals with chronic diseases e.g. diabetes, arthritis.

Men and women's health

Women's health

Women live on average longer than men but have higher rates of hospital admission and consultation with their GP than men. This is partly explained by pregnancy and childbirth, but there are clear differences between the genders in the causes of morbidity and mortality. Population surveys indicate that women prefer to have a choice when it comes to the gender of doctor they consult (Preston-Whyte et al 1983). Studies in general practice have also shown that both men and women choose to consult a doctor of their own gender not only for sex-specific disorders, but also for conditions that are not sex linked.

Although certain diseases, for example cervical neoplasia and endometriosis, affect only women, the most common causes of mortality are similar to those seen in men, namely cardiovascular disease and lung cancer.

Finally, women are prescribed drugs more often and for a longer period of time than men. They are in particular 2–3 times more likely to have been prescribed psychotropic medications (hypnotics, tranquillisers or antidepressants) than men. Moreover, women are also more likely to have taken non-prescription medicines than men. The explanations for these phenomena are not clear, involving patient and doctor factors, culture, marketing and history.

This section will highlight some of the key issues related to women's health, ranging from health promotion to specific diseases.

Health promotion

This is now a key component of everyday general practice, accounting for up to 20% of GPs' time. It involves three overlapping activities (Tannahill 1985):

1. health education
2. the prevention of ill-health
3. health protection.

Health promotion is particularly relevant for women because it addresses not only their personal needs, but also the needs of those for whom many women act as carers, that is, children and older relatives. GPs are often greatly assisted in this work by other members of the primary health-care team, particularly health visitors, practice nurses, midwives and community nurses. As well as offering health promotion advice on an opportunistic basis during routine consultations, many practices also run well-woman clinics.

Areas that offer considerable opportunities for health promotion include cervical and breast screening, contraception, smoking and drinking.

Cervical screening

Cervical cancer is the eighth most common cancer in women, 84% of new cases of invasive cancer occurring in women aged 35 and over. However, 87% of cases of cervical carcinoma in situ (the pre-malignant phase) occur in women aged under 45. Known risk factors include sexual behaviour, infection with human papilloma virus, cigarette smoking, pregnancy at an early age, a lower socio-economic status and a history of dyskaryosis. There is controversy over the possible role of oral contraceptives, but barrier methods seem to provide a protective effect.

Cervical screening programmes have been operating in the UK for over 30 years, but a national standardised, computerised call and recall programme was not introduced until the mid-1980s. Cervical screening is currently recommended for all sexually active women aged 20–64, regular smears being taken every 3–5 years. The aim of the programme is to identify and treat abnormalities that might otherwise develop into invasive cancer. Cervical intra-epithelial neoplasia (CIN) is a general term covering a range of abnormalities (Table 1).

Well over 80% of women have normal cervical smears, 5–10% of all smears being inadequate (usually because of technical reasons) and needing to be repeated. Between 4% and 5% show borderline or mild dyskaryosis (CIN1), and 1.5–2.0% moderate or severe dyskaryosis (CIN2 or 3). A single borderline or mildly dyskaryotic smear should be repeated in 6 months. If the changes persist, referral for colposcopy is recommended for all patients whose smears show moderate or severe dyskaryosis.

Breast screening

Breast cancer is the most common malignancy in women, accounting for 21% of all new female cases. The overall lifetime risk of developing the disease is 1 in 11. Known risk factors include a family history, an early onset of the menarche, alcohol and exposure to ionising radiation. Breast-feeding, early menopause and an early full-term pregnancy have a protective effect.

Since 1991 there has been a national breast screening programme offering 3 yearly mammography to all women aged 50–64; there is no currently no evidence that routine mammography in women under 50 years old is of any benefit. About 70–80% of screen-detected cancers have a good prognosis.

GPs and other primary care health professionals are well placed to encourage their patients to attend for mammography.

Other cancers

In women the next most common cancers are those of the large bowel, lung, ovary and uterus.

Contraception

Advice on contraception is readily available from GPs, health visitors, practice nurses, midwives, community nurses and family planning clinics. The popularity of different methods of contraception varies over time, influenced partly by fashion and partly by health scares. The trends in usage between 1976 and 1989 are shown in Table 2.

Decisions about the choice of contraceptive method depend on a variety of factors – personal and partner preferences, age, religion, culture/ethnicity, family and personal

Table 1 Cervical intra-epithelial neoplasia (CIN)		
Cytology	**CIN grade**	**Histology**
Mild dyskaryosis	1	Mild dysplasia
Moderate dyskaryosis	2	Moderate dysplasia
Severe dyskaryosis	3	Severe dysplasia and carcinoma in situ

Table 2 Trends in contraceptive use in Great Britain 1976, 1983, 1986 and 1989 in women aged 18–44

Current usual method of contraception	Survey			
	FFS[1] 1976	GHS[2] 1983	GHS 1986	GHS 1989
	%			
Users[3]	68	75	75	72
Pill	29	28	26	25
IUD	6	6	8	6
Condom	14	13	13	16
Cap	2	1	2	1
Withdrawal	5	4	4	4
Safe period	1	1	2	2
Other	1	1	1	1
Female sterilization	7	11	11	11
Male sterilization	6	10	12	12
Non-users	31	25	25	28
Sterile after another operation	2	2	2	3
Pregnant/wanting to get pregnant	7	7	8	9
Abstinence/no partner	– } 23	– } 16	12 } 16	14 } 18
Other	–	–	4	4
Base = 100%[4]	5231	4444	4879	4776

[1]FFS = Family Formation Survey. [2]GHS = General Household Survey. [3]Abstinence is not included as a method of contraception. Those who said 'going without sex to avoid getting pregnant' was their only method of contraception are shown with 'others' as not using a method. [4]Percentages add to more than 100 because some women used more than one method or had more than one reason for not using a method.

Source: McPherson (1993)

Table 3 User-failure rates for different methods of contraception per 100 woman-years (1991)

	Range in the world literature[1]	Oxford/FPA Study[2] – all women married and aged above 25		
		Overall (any duration)	Age 25–34 (≤2 years use)	Age 35+ (≤2 years use)
Sterilisation				
Male (after azzospermia)	0–0.05	0.02	0.08	0.08
Female	0–0.5	0.13	0.45	0.08
Subcutaneous implant				
(Jadelle)	0–0.1			
Implanton	0–0.07			
Injectable (DMPA)	0–1.0	–	–	–
Combined pills				
50 µg oestrogen	0.1–3	0.16	0.25	0.17
<50 µg oestrogen	0.2–3	0.27	0.38	0.23
Progestogen-only pill	0.3–4	1.2	2.5	0.5
IUD				
Nova-T/Multiload Cu 250	1–2			
Nova-T380	0.6			
Multiload Cu 375	0.2–1			
Cu-T380	0.2–1			
Levonorgestrel IUD-20	0.1–0.2			
Diaphragm	4–20	1.9	5.5	2.8
(Male) Condom	2–15	3.6	6.0	2.9
Female condom	5–15			
Coitus interruptus	6–17	6.7	–	–
Spermicides alone	4–25	11.9	–	–
Fertility awareness	2–25	15.5	–	–
'Persona'	6–?	–	–	–
No method, young women	80–90	–	–	–
No method at age 40	40–50	–	–	–
No method at age 45	10–20	–	–	–
No method at age 50 (if still having menses)	0–5	–	–	–

[1]Excludes atypical studies giving particularly poor results and all extended-use studies. For sterilization, rates in first column (only) are *lifetime failure rates*.
[2]Lancet report in 1982.

Notes: 1. First figure of ranges in first column gives a rough measure of 'perfect use' (but is not the same).
2. Influence of age: all the rates in the fourth column being lower than those in the third column. Lower rates still to be expected above age 45.
3. Much better results obtainable in other states of relative infertility, such as lactation.
4. Oxford/FPA users were established users at recruitment – greatly improving results for barrier methods.

Source: Guillebaud (1999)

medical history, parity and the need for reliability. The user-failure rates for different methods of contraception are shown in Table 3.

Smoking and drinking

The rate of decline in cigarette smoking over the past 25 years has been greater in men than in women, the proportion of smokers in both genders now being virtually the same. Recently, however, there has been an increase in the number of young women taking up smoking. The risk of a heart attack, a stroke or other cardiovascular disease is increased tenfold in young women taking oral contraceptives, and is even greater in women aged over 45. Cigarette smoking is also linked to low birthweight and an increased risk of CIN and invasive cancer.

Women are more sensitive to alcohol than are men, partly because of differences in their weight and body composition (as women have proportionately less water in their bodies than men). Moreover, oral contraceptives cause a slowing of alcohol metabolism, resulting in a delayed elimination of alcohol from the blood, with implications for car drivers. As with smoking, there is evidence of an increase in the number of young women taking up drinking and exceeding the recommended 'safe' limits (14 units per week compared with 21 units for men).

In addition to the physical and psychological problems associated with excessive alcohol consumption, pregnant women are at risk of producing babies with fetal alcohol syndrome, a condition involving microcephaly, developmental delay, growth deficiency and characteristic facial and limb anomalies.

Benign breast disease

Breast problems are relatively common in general practice, with an annual incidence of 30 per 1000 women. The majority of these patients fortunately have benign conditions, cancer being diagnosed in only about 6% of symptomatic referrals. The most frequent presenting symptoms are:

- lumps
- pain
- nipple discharge
- nipple retraction or distortion.

The incidence of benign breast conditions and cancer varies with age (Fig. 1, see p. 48).

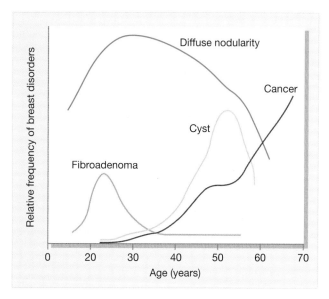

Fig. 1 **Incidence of breast cancer and benign breast conditions against age.**
Source: Austoker et al (1999). Reproduced with permission from NHS Breast Screening Programme

Menstrual problems

Menstrual disorders fall in the top 10 most common specific conditions presenting in general practice and are the second most frequent cause of overall hospital referral, irrespective of the patient's age or gender. A variety of disorders can present:

- excessive bleeding (menorrhagia)
- no bleeding (amenorrhoea)
- too-frequent bleeding (polymenorrhoea)
- infrequent bleeding (oligomenorrhoea)
- painful bleeding (dysmenorrhoea)
- intermenstrual bleeding
- post-coital bleeding
- post-menopausal bleeding.

Careful history-taking and examination are required to identify the underlying gynaecological, endocrine or haematological causes.

Menopause

The menopause is the time at which menstruation ceases, the average age at which this occurs being just over 50. The climacteric is the period of gradual ovarian failure, lasting several years, that precedes the menopause.

Symptoms associated with the climacteric are common, but only about 25% of women seek medical advice. Problems associated with the climacteric and menopause include:

- vasomotor symptoms, hot flushes and night sweats
- menstrual changes – prolonged, irregular or heavy periods
- psychological problems – emotional lability, depression and poor concentration
- sexual problems – loss of libido and dyspareunia

- genitourinary problems – frequency, urgency, stress incontinence and vaginal dryness
- musculoskeletal problems – muscle and joint pains
- cardiovascular disease – occurring 10–15 years post-menopausally
- osteoporosis – seen 10–15 years post menopause.

The successful management of symptoms involves psychological support, life-style (smoking, diet, and exercise) advice and medication, both hormonal and non-hormonal. For those patients requiring hormone replacement therapy (HRT), unopposed continuous oestrogen can be given to women who have had a hysterectomy, but cyclical oestrogen–progestogen therapy is required for those who still possess a uterus. However, in the light of the recently published Women's Health Initiative trial in the USA, the prolonged (i.e. more than 5 years) use of oral oestrogen plus progestin HRT is not recommended. For every 10 000 women taking this prolonged HRT there would be eight more pulmonary emboli (2.13-fold increase), eight more strokes (1.41-fold increase), eight more breast cancers (1.26-fold increase) and seven more myocardial infarcts (1.29-fold increase) each year. However, there would also be six fewer bowel cancers (0.63-fold decrease) and five fewer hip fractures (0.66-fold decrease) each year. For those women who have been on combined oral HRT for more than 5 years, risk factors, past medical and family history and personal preferences will need to be considered before a decision to continue or withdraw therapy is made.

Men's health

Men and their health

Doctors see men at the extremes of life but men are largely absent from the health care environment from their adolescence until the late middle age. Research has shown that men do not feel vulnerable when it comes to their health. Men have a sense of being in control of their health and also a need to be in control. Attending a doctor often means handing over control of their lives or their bodies. Risk taking seems to be a normal part of development for men which if carried out in sport can be reasonable safe, but there are many tragic examples of risk taking on the roads, with drugs and with alcohol. Risk taking has inevitable health consequences that are minimised in men's minds because of their feeling of invulnerability.

Take-up in prevention programmes is less for men than for women. Those men with higher education and social class levels have better uptakes and many men attend because of the influence of their spouse. Men's knowledge about their health can be quite poor: a MORI poll asked men about the location of their prostates and 13% of men could correctly identify its location while 16% of women identified correctly.

In general practice men are often apologetic when they attend and are willing to see locums as they seem not to value a doctor–patient relationship in the same way as women. Males are often absent in therapy such as family therapy, family and relationship therapy, and counselling.

When it comes to taking a history from men, it is important to remember that they may be poor at disclosing and remembering information. They are also slower to act on physical symptoms and most shrewd general practitioners listen carefully to the symptoms of a middle-aged male whom they have not seen for some time.

Men seem to be willing to attend the Accident and Emergency department (A & E) and 50% of attendees at A & E are male. Similarly, men will avail of primary care in the workplace even though there may be confidentiality issues that need to be clarified, as the doctor running such a service may have a primary loyalty and responsibility to the employer and not to the patient.

Infant mortality is about 20% higher for males than females, and males have a higher death rate for each age group throughout life. Life expectancy has increased for both males and females, but it is still lower in men than in women, being 73 years for the average man and 78 years for the average woman. The four main causes of premature death in men are:

1. diseases of the circulatory system
2. cancer
3. accidents
4. suicide.

Ischaemic heart disease (Fig. 2) accounts for about 70% of the circulatory disease deaths. Lung cancer accounts for about 25% of deaths from neoplasms, and over 60% of accidental deaths occur in car accidents. The rate of suicide increases with age in men.

The fourth national morbidity study chronicles the details of 500 000 people who attend their GP. It reveals interesting gender differences, females in the 14–64 year age group consulting more frequently for all diseases and conditions than males (Fig. 3), the study excluding routine antenatal care. Men consult their GP less often for genitourinary disease, mental disorders, blood diseases and ill-defined conditions. The differences in such a consulting pattern do not, however, mean that men are any healthier: Table 2 shows illnesses with a twofold excess in men. Table 2 predictably shows excesses in the area of cardiovascular disease, gout, venereal disease and alcohol dependence.

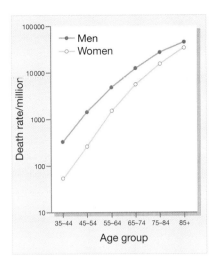

Fig. 2 **Deaths from ischaemic heart disease, England and Wales, 1991.** (Men's Health Fig. 1.3 p 9)

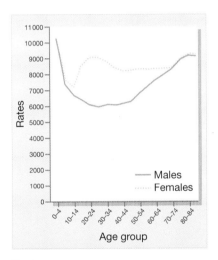

Fig. 3 **Variation in consulting rate (per 10 000 person–years at risk) between men and women for all diseases and conditions.**

Risk modification

There are three areas in which risk modification is of proven value:

■ stopping smoking
■ identifying and treating raised blood pressure
■ reducing alcohol intake.

Stopping smoking

Giving up smoking is probably the single most important step that a man can take to improve his health. Over half of all men who smoke want to stop, but most believe that it is not possible. Smokers present to their GP with more instances of upper and lower respiratory tract infection, angina and myocardial infarction. Smokers will also be identified during checks at well-man clinics. The attendance at such clinics is variable, however, with a high rate of non-attendance. Identifying those who are interested in giving up smoking is a useful start. Prochaska and Di Clemente's (1992) readiness to change model is helpful to smokers who may not be considering change (pre-contemplation), who are considering it (contemplation) or who are ready to change. The provision of information support and nicotine replacement increases the chances of staying abstinent. The success rate is still, however, modest: only 10% still not smoking 1 year later.

Hypertension

Hypertension is another major cause of cardiovascular disease and strokes. Men may present to their GP having diagnosed themselves or been diagnosed at work. The GP may also identify hypertensives through opportunistic case-finding when the patient presents for something entirely different. As a diagnosis of hypertension has lifelong implications, it should be made only after repeated checking of the blood pressure over a 3–4 week period.

A modification of the diet, particularly in terms of fat and salt reduction, and weight loss are important parts of the management strategy. Numerous medications exist for the treatment of hypertension, and hospitals and GPs are increasingly agreeing on joint protocols for the management of hypertension. Such treatments are always based on cost-effective pharmacological preparations with a low side-effect profile.

Table 2 Rates of patients consulting per 1000 persons at risk per year

	M	F	Ratio (M/F)
Other venereal disease	0.8	0.3	2.67
Malignant neoplasm of bladder	0.6	0.2	3.00
Gout	6.4	1.6	4.00
Sexual deviations and disorders	2.3	0.8	2.88
Alcohol dependence syndrome	2	0.6	3.33
Acute myocardial infarction	*3.8*	*2*	*1.90*
Old myocardial infarction	0.9	0.3	3.00
Angina pectoris	*13*	*9.8*	*1.33*
Other forms of chronic ischaemic heart disease	*6.2*	*3.3*	*1.88*
Aortic aneurysm	0.5	0.1	5.00
Deflected nasal septum	0.8	0.3	2.67
Nasal polyps	1.1	0.5	2.20
Emphysema	1.1	0.5	2.20
Duodenal ulcer	4.6	2.1	2.19
Inguinal hernia	5.7	0.6	9.50
Abscess of anal and rectal regions	1	0.4	2.50
Congenital anomalies of genital organs	1.3	0.1	13.00

NB: Episode rates given to nearest integer, ratios to two decimal places

Alcohol

Men can in general drink up to three or four units of alcohol a day without compromising their health. However, a quarter of men drink over the daily recommended benchmark, which can lead to:

- an increase in blood pressure
- weight gain
- a long-term risk of heart disease
- cancer of the mouth, throat or oesophagus
- liver and brain damage.

However, for men over 40 years of age, drinking two to three units of red wine daily has a protective effect against cardiovascular disease.

Excessive drinking can be difficult to pick up in general practice before it leads to health problems, but asking patients about their alcohol intake and providing information about sensible drinking does make a difference. Almost all road traffic accidents in males involve recent alcohol ingestion.

Urological problems

It is in the area of urology that doctors deal with problems that are unique to men. Men's knowledge of their own genitourinary system is, however, poor.

Prostate conditions

The prostate is a small gland encircling the upper part of the urethra. It produces a milky, alkaline secretion that accounts for up to a third of the semen volume and plays a role in activating sperm. The prostate gland is a common site of pathology in elderly men, yet a 1995 MORI poll found that only 13% of men could correctly identify its location.

Benign prostatic hyperplasia

The bulk of prostatic disease is caused by benign prostatic hypertrophy, which increases with age until about 80% of men over the age of 80 have hyperplasia. Its symptoms are divided into:

- *obstructive symptoms* caused by constriction of the urethra by the enlarged prostate, these include hesitancy, a weak stream, straining, prolonged micturition, a feeling of incomplete bladder emptying and overflow incontinence
- *irritative symptoms* caused by an irritable bladder muscle secondary to high voiding pressures and incomplete emptying, symptoms include nocturia, daytime frequency, urgency and urge incontinence.

In men with mild-to-moderate prostatic symptoms, a watch-and-wait policy is reasonable as such men are unlikely to develop serious complications. Men with obstructive symptoms are significantly more likely than those with irritative symptoms to need a prostatectomy.

Surgical options include prostatectomy and transuretheral resection of the prostate. Alpha-adrenergic blocking agents that act on the bladder neck to inhibit myocontractility are useful advances. A second group of drugs that can arrest or reverse prostatic growth manipulate the hormone testosterone by converting it into dihydrotestosterone.

Prostatic carcinoma

This disease is found in as many as 50% of men over the age of 70 years, but it is now occurring in an increasing number of men between the ages of 45 and 65. If detected early enough, the disease is potentially curable. Diagnosis is, however, difficult, and the traditional rectal examination has poor sensitivity and specificity. Much interest has focused on prostatic-specific antigen, a tumour marker used to measure the response of prostatic cancer to treatment. On its own, it has low sensitivity, which means that the prostate-specific antigen level may be raised in disease-negative men. Transrectal ultrasonography is increasingly being used, although this may also miss up to 40% of cases. The symptoms of prostatic cancer may mimic those of benign prostatic hypertrophy, although prostatic cancer is a much less common condition in general practice. There is currently a lack of evidence as to whether screening for prostate cancer actually offers benefits to offset its obvious harms.

Testicular cancer

The incidence of testicular cancer has almost doubled in the past 28 years in populations in England and Wales (Power et al 2001). The incidence of teratomas is maximal at about 30 years of age, whereas for seminomas it is maximum at 40. Patients are increasingly presenting with a fear of testicular cancer.

Patients with testicular cancer may present with a change in size or weight of one testicle. However, one testicle is often a little larger than the other, but changes need careful assessment. A dull ache in the scrotum, groin or lower back is also important. It is important to diagnose testicular cancer early as survival after diagnosis and treatment is good. With an increasing interest in men's health, the promotion of testicular self-examination is increasing the number of young men consulting the GP, which will hopefully be translated into better diagnosis and an increased survival rate.

Erectile problems

These can affect up to 10% of the adult male population, the incidence increasing with age. The causes of erectile function are divided into physical (Table 3) and emotional (Table 4). Physical causes are now thought to be commoner than emotional causes and many are remediable to treatment and advice.

What can make a difference?

Most men know that smoking is bad for them and helping men to give up smoking with information and nicotine replacement has long-term cardiovascular and respiratory benefits. Similarly, identifying and treating raised blood pressures is important, especially in reducing the incidence of cerebrovascular accidents.

Alcohol consumption can gradually increase in men and merely asking about alcohol intake and informing them that 28 units per week is a safe limit is helpful. Alcohol has other adverse metabolic and psychological effects, which can be improved by drinking within safe limits. The management of proven circulatory diseases is important and there is strong evidence that having a reminder system for chronic disease is effective in its ongoing management for both men and women.

Table 3 **Physical causes of impotence**
■ Alcohol
■ Drug misuse
■ Side-effects of medication
■ Circulatory disorders
■ Chronic physical disease
■ Neurological diseases

Table 4 **Emotional causes of impotence**
■ Fear of failure
■ Unexpressed anger
■ Sadness resulting from the loss of a partner after many years of marriage
■ Guilt about sexual desires being seen as perverted, dirty or shameful

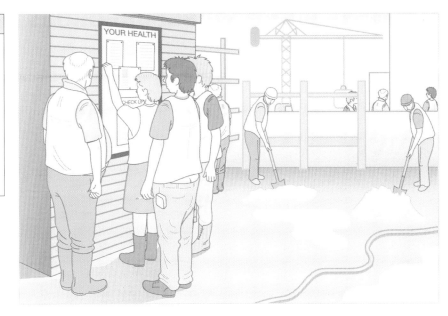

Fig. 3 **The work place can be a good venue for offering health advice to men.**

Box 1 A Wellman check
Family history
Alcohol
Exercise
Smoking
Nutrition
Blood pressure
Lipids
Urinalysis
Body mass index
Urinary symptoms

Sadly, many men with benign prostatic hypertrophy end up in A & E with acute retention of urine. Informing men about benign prostatic hypertrophy and engaging in active and planned management of the disorder is of considerable benefit to the quality of life.

Diagnosis of depression in men can be difficult as it may present with undue aggression, causing violence and road traffic accidents. However, the response to treatment for men is excellent.

Offering health checks

A general practitioner's surgery may not be the best place to offer health promotion to men. On the other hand work is a good venue as there is some evidence that men will avail of workplace opportunities to have health checks and advice. Great care has to be taken that the process is confidential and that it has the confidence of employees and their unions. Health and safety checks have been offered to made workers on building sites and in offices. Attempts are occasionally made to offer health advice to men in social settings such as all-male clubs and in pubs. The success of such ventures need to be managed carefully as alcohol is likely to be a major distraction.

Conventional wisdom in the popular media indicates that men are not interested in their health and are all too willing to engage in risky and unhealthy behaviours. In countries where the patient has to pay the doctor, men will postpone seeing the doctor in favour of another family member. In a Dublin practice 25% of middle-aged men postponed seeing the doctor because of consultation charges. Other barriers also exist, such as lack of time, shift work and limited access.

Men engage in risk in both work and sport and it seems to be an important part of engagement and enjoyment. Harm reduction, rather than prohibition or prevention, can reduce risk to sensible proportions through health and safety training, adequate training and the use of good, safe and serviced equipment in both work and play.

Men and women's health

- Women live longer than men but have higher rates of hospital admission and GP consultation than men.
- There are clear differences in morbidity and mortality between women and men.
- Women consume more drugs, especially psychotropic medications, than men.
- Health promotion involves health education, the prevention of ill-health and health protection
- Men are often absent from the health care services.
- Men may be poor at remembering and disclosing information
- Men die 5 years earlier than women.
- Main causes of premature death are, cardiovascular disease, cancer, accidents and suicide.
- Even with nicotine replacement only 10% will have stopped smoking a year later.
- One quarter of men drink over the limit of 21 units per week.
- Testicular cancer, a disease of younger men has almost doubled over the last 25 years.

Acute respiratory tract infections

These constitute about 25% of the work of general practice and account for nearly one third of admissions to hospital. Acute respiratory tract infections account for one third of all consultations between doctor and child.

In children, most infections affect the upper respiratory tract, comprising the ears, nose and throat. The overall incidence of acute respiratory infections peaks in early childhood and declines with age. Parental smoking increases the risk of all respiratory illnesses in children, the risk being greater in infants than in older children. Exposure to other children or adults also increases the chance of infection, crèche, playschool and school attendance providing powerful vectors for respiratory tract illness. Children who are breast-fed have fewer infections than those who are not, which is presumed to be related to an immune-mediated protective effect of breast milk.

Over 90% of respiratory tract infections are caused by viruses, most by rhinoviruses (30–50%) and coronaviruses (5–20%), the remainder by influenza, parainfluenza and adeno-respiratory syncytial and entericviruses. Respiratory syncytial virus causes up to 80% of cases of bronchiolitis and 15% of those of croup.

Bacteria

These account for a much lower proportion of lower respiratory tract infections in children than in adults. Gram-negative organisms and group B beta-haemolytic streptococci are the most common bacterial pathogens encountered in the newborn, whereas *Haemophilus influenzae* and *Staphylococcus aureus* are important in infants.

Croup

This is the most common cause of acute airways obstruction in children, presenting as inspiratory stridor, barking cough, hoarseness and varying degrees of respiratory distress. Viral croup accounts for over 95% of cases and spread is by droplets and by direct contact. The dramatic presentation of symptoms can be alarming, especially for new parents. Fortunately, most cases can be managed at home with the help of a steam kettle and/or a steamy bathroom, an avoidance of smoking and antipyretics if necessary (Fig. 1).

The common cold

This is caused by a number of viral agents, 40% being rhinoviruses, 15% coronaviruses and the remainder parainfluenza, influenza and respiratory syncitical viruses. It is transmitted via droplet spread and hand, mouth and nose contact. The incubation period is between 1 and 3 days, the risk of infection being higher for smokers; crowded environments and psychological stress also increase susceptibility. The common cold presents as a runny nose, sore throat, hoarseness and a cough. Complications include sinusitis, otitis media and acute lower respiratory tract infections in susceptible individuals.

Symptomatic relief is the order of the day while the common cold runs its course. Patients are increasingly accepting of the fact that antibiotics do not have a role to play in an uncomplicated common cold.

Acute pharyngitis/tonsilitis

Most cases are viral in origin, a minority being streptococcal. The presence of white exudate on the tonsil is not a reliable guide to the presence of a bacterial infection even though it is often used by GPs as a reason for prescribing. Patients present with acute sore throat; many will feel clammy, and a few will have a fever. Systemic symptoms include loss of appetite, headache, myalgia and malaise. It is common to find cervical lymphadenopathy, and pharyngitis can also cause pain referred to the ear.

It is worth taking a throat swab in patients with recurrent infections, and many GPs will treat patients with tonsillar exudate and systemic symptoms using a 7 day course of penicillin. Most patients will, however, obtain sufficient pain relief and improvement of their symptoms with aspirin or paracetamol gargles and regular fluid intake. The general rule of '3 days coming, 3 days there and 3 days disappearing' is useful in advising patients about prognosis.

Young adults may present with a massive exudative tonsilitis and severe systemic symptoms together with generalised lymphadenopathy, hepatitis, splenomegaly and a thrombocytopaenia on full blood count. The patient may also complain of a rash since taking amoxicillin earlier in the illness. This illness is nowadays known as Epstein–Barr viral-associated infectious mononucleosis, although it used to be known as 'kissing disease' because of the proposed mode of transmission. A full blood count will reveal an atypical mononucleosis and the presence of red cell antibodies, this being known as a positive monospot result. The condition often presents in students prior to examinations, and steroids often produce a dramatic response within 48 hours.

Sinusitis

This presents as nasal congestion, runny nose, fever, pain, and tenderness over the maxillary sinuses. The patient occasionally experiences pain on

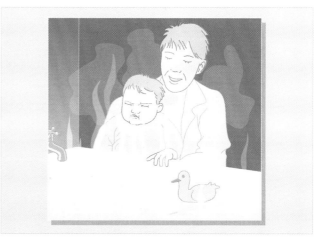

Fig. 1 **Viral croup – most cases can be treated at home using steam.**

coughing or bending forwards, which points to ethmoidal sinusitis. Predisposing factors include a deviated nasal septum, polyps and smoking, and pollution.

Causative agents include aerobic bacteria such as *Streptococcus pneumonia* and *H. influenzae* and anaerobic organisms such as *bacteroides*. Viruses including rhino-viruses, parainfluenza and adeno-viruses, can be isolated in up to 15% of patients with sinusitis.

Management includes menthol inhalation to assist the drainage of the sinuses and antibiotics such as amoxicillin or erythromycin.

Otitis media
This may present as an inflamed tympanic membrane with or without a middle ear effusion. The tympanic membrane occasionally bursts, leading to a purulent discharge and consequent easing of the pain. The predominant symptom is that of earache, with irritability and fever. Although its peak incidence is in early childhood, otitis media is still common in adults. The Eustachian tube is shorter in children than in adults and seems to be less effective in protecting the middle ear from ascending infection from the nasopharynx as well as in draining the contents of the middle ear into the nasopharynx. Acute otitis media is more common in children with a cleft palate, in those in poor socio-economic circumstances and in those exposed to tobacco smoke; breast-fed children seem to have a lower incidence. Both viruses and bacteria have been implicated in otitis media in almost equal amount. Rhinoviruses and respiratory syncytial virus have been the most common pathogens isolated, whereas *Strep. pneumoniae*, *H. influenzae* and *Moxarella catarrhalis* are the most common bacterial pathogens.

There is a high rate of natural resolution in acute otitis media, but few doctors withhold antibiotics from such patients. Amoxycillin is a commonly prescribed antibiotic for otitis media.

Lower respiratory tract infections
The most common of these are acute bronchitis and pneumonia.

Acute bronchitis
Acute bronchitis is an inflammation of the bronchii that is more common in smokers and occurs more frequently in the winter months. It causes an acute cough usually productive of yellow/green sputum that may occasionally be blood stained. The patient may have a raised temperature, with night sweats and fatigue. Shortness of breath on effort is noticeable, and wheezing may also be present.

Risk factors include cigarette smoke, passive smoking, air pollution, overcrowded living conditions and being in a lower socio-economic group. Bacterial causes include *H. influenzae*, *Strep. pneumoniae* and *Branhamella catarrhalis*. Viruses include respiratory syncytial viruses, influenza and parainfluenza viruses, together with rhinoviruses and adenoviruses. Chest signs include basal crepitations and some expiratory wheezing.

Most GPs treat acute bronchitis empirically with amoxycillin or erythromycin. The illness provides an opportunity to advise on cigarette-smoking or occupational dusts and gases.

Pneumonia
Pneumonia is a lung infection showing involvement of the alveoli, with a resulting consolidation of the alveolar air spaces. It is the consolidation that distinguishes pneumonia from bronchitis, which involves only the airway mucosa and walls. The term 'community-acquired pneumonia' is now widely used to distinguish it from the pneumonias acquired in hospital from the unusual range of organisms present there.

Community-acquired pneumonia can range from a mild infection, like a bronchitis, to a life-threatening illness needing hospitalisation. As much pneumonia goes undiagnosed and even unreported providing a true incidence is difficult. It is, however, estimated that the incidence of lower respiratory tract infections is 44 per 1000 patients per year, and that of community-acquired pneumonia probably 10–12 cases per 1000 per year.

A practice of 2000 patients can therefore expect to see up to 20 cases per year.

The organisms most common implicated in pneumonia are *Strep. pneumoniae*, *H. influenzae* and *Legionella*, the most common non-bacterial cause being *Mycoplasma pneumoniae*.

Most patients present with malaise and fever, and there may be symptoms of lung and pleuritic pain. Cough is almost universally present, as is breathlessness. To demonstrate dullness to percussion and increased vocal resonance, there needs to be a substantial area of consolidation. Coarse crackles are, however, commonly heard, a wheeze being less common. Sputum culture and a chest X-ray are the basis of confirmatory diagnosis in the community. Antibiotic therapy with amoxicillin or erythromycin is the mainstay of management for non-severe community-acquired pneumonia.

Pollution
There is considerable evidence in both the USA and in Europe showing that long-term exposure to pollution is associated with increased mortality from respiratory and cardiovascular disease and lung cancer. The main pollutants are particulate matter in black smoke, nitrogen dioxide and sulphur dioxide. Several studies have shown that chronic respiratory disease in children is associated with air pollution and it is now well recognised that the incidence of cardio-pulmonary disease is increased the nearer the patient lives to the pollutated street or highway. The adjusted death rates for respiratory deaths in Dublin declined by 15.5% following a ban on coal sales in 1990. Doctors practising in heavily congested urban environments are likely to see much acute and chronic respiratory illnesses, which will reduce with reduction in emissions from coal and petrol. Emission control will, however, need to be pursued at local, national and international levels.

Acute respiratory tract infections
- Acute respiratory tract illnesses account for one-third of all consultations between the GP and a child.
- Over 90% of respiratory tract infections are caused by viruses.
- Croup is an acute airways obstruction in children which can be managed at home with the help of a steam kettle.
- Lower respiratory tract illnesses such as acute bronchitis and pneumonia are mainly treated with antibiotics.
- Patients living in polluted environments suffer much more acute and chronic respiratory tract illness.

Gastrointestinal infections

Sudden attacks of diarrhoea, with or without vomiting, are usually due to infections of the digestive system, although they can be due to direct poisoning from toxic chemicals in food or (particularly in the very young and the very old) a sign of more serious kinds of illness (such as twisting of the bowel in babies, or cancer in the elderly).

Common causes
Infections, so-called *gastro-enteritis*, are very common (Box 1). Essentially, the infections are passed on through the faeces, which is why the most important advice in prevention is to wash hands thoroughly after defaecation and before handling foodstuffs (Box 2). An infected person involved in preparing food for others can pass infections on to large numbers of people very quickly, and this is the usual cause of large outbreaks.

Symptoms
The most common infections are viral or bacterial (Boxes 3 and 4) and, although they may cause very unpleasant, even incapacitating, symptoms they generally are not a serious threat to health, last for only a few days at most and go away spontaneously without any treatment. However, the human body is comprised mostly of fluid and loss of this is the main threat to health. In very hot climates, the loss of fluid can be accelerated, but more important is the proportionately greater effect of fluid loss on babies and, to a lesser extent, the elderly.

Treatment
Replacement of body fluid is the key treatment in all cases, usually simply by drinking more than usual. Although some of the bacterial infections (the commonest in UK are *Salmonella* and *Campylobacter*, originating mostly from eggs and poultry products) could be treated with antibiotics, these are not generally needed and may even prolong the time that a person is infected so that they pass the infection on to even more people.

Rare but serious infections
There are a few potentially very serious intestinal infections which are,

---

Box 1

It is estimated that there are over nine million cases of gastrointestinal infection every year in England and Wales with 300 deaths and 35 000 hospital admissions. Accurate figures are difficult to compile because most cases are minor and do not need medical attention.

Source: Wheeler et al 1999

Box 2 Prevention of gastrointestinal infections – food hygiene

- Persons who have recently had possible gastrointestinal infection should not handle food for others
- Cuts and grazes on the hands should be covered when handling food
- Raw food and cooked food should not come into contact. Separate cutting boards and other equipment should be used and they should be stored separately in refrigerators etc.
- Pets should not be allowed to come into contact with food to be eaten by humans and hands should be washed after contact with pets
- Hands should be washed frequently whilst handling food, between handling raw and cooked food and before eating
- Some foods e.g. minced or processed beef, chicken, eggs and pork, need to be particularly thoroughly cooked all the way through because they are likely to contain harmful bacteria that need to be destroyed by cooking
- Dishcloths, hand towels etc are a frequent cause of cross-contamination. Paper towels are better
- Perishable food, especially leftovers, should be thrown away if there is any doubt about storage e.g. if it has been left out of the refrigerator for more than an hour or so
- Cooked food should not be re-heated more than once and should always be thoroughly heated right through the food
- Pregnant women should not eat pate and certain soft cheeses e.g. Brie and Camembert because of the danger of listeria contamination which might affect the pregnancy

This is not an exhaustive list of advice about food hygiene but contains most of the important points. The UK Goverment's Food Standards Agency has an excellent website (www.food.gov.uk) giving detailed advice and information for the public.

Adapted from Forbes (1996)

Box 3 Main organisms that cause gastro-enteritis

Bacteria

- *Campylobacter*
- *Salmonella*
- *Clostridium perfringens*
- *Listeria*
- *E. coli*

Viruses

- Norwalk-like viruses, rotavirus and other viruses (see Box 4)

Adapted from Food Standards Agency Website www.food.gov.uk

---

fortunately, not very common in the UK and other developed countries. The most important include one particular variety of *E. coli* – a bacteria which is universally found in the faeces of all animals including humans. Most types are harmless but *E. coli* 0152 can cause very serious infections in vulnerable people such as children and the elderly, with unusual general effects on the body which can in some cases result in kidney failure and death (Box 5). Other kinds of more serious infections, such as typhoid and cholera, both of which may also kill vulnerable people, still occur in underdeveloped countries.

Increased worldwide travel greatly increases the potential for spread of infections from one country to another. 'Traveller's diarrhoea' has become accepted as an inevitability of foreign holidays. Most of the time it is not due to potentially serious infections, but there is always that possibility. Travellers from developed countries like UK are advised to protect themselves against infection by such measures as being immunised against serious infections like typhoid and cholera, if necessary; scrupulous handwashing; and being careful to avoid drinking possibly contaminated water (even through ice-cubes or tooth-brushing) or food (particularly uncooked food).

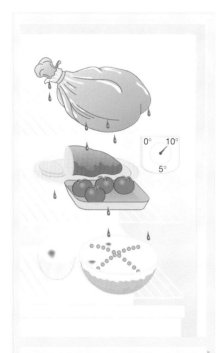

- Raw meat should be stored in sealable containers at the bottom of the fridge
- Keep food at the right temperature
- Observe 'use by' dates

Fig. 1 **The correct storage of food is important in the prevention of gastrointestinal infection.**

Box 4 **Foodborne virus infections**

Most of these infections are caused by Norwalk-like viruses, which used to be known as small round structured viruses (SRSV). This is a group of viruses, including Hawaii, Snow Mountain, Taunton, Mexico and Grimsby viruses, which appear to cause an identical picture of projectile vomiting and diarrhoea. The names are derived from where they were first identified, but they are difficult to detect routinely and not much is known about them. The infection is thought to be spread mainly through contamination of food during preparation by food handlers who are already infected with the virus. These viruses are also found in shellfish, especially oysters, which are usually eaten raw, whereas cooking of other types of shellfish will usually destroy any virus contamination. The contamination of shellfish results from them filtering large volumes of seawater during feeding. As they are usually harvested from inshore coastal waters, this water can contain sewage contaminated by the viruses. Although well diluted in the seawater, the shellfish in effect filter the virus out of large quantities of water. This is one reason why sewage contamination needs to be reduced in coastal waters, particularly in shellfish harvesting areas.

Based on Hale A 1999 Foodborne viral infections. BMJ; 318: 1433–4

Box 5 **Examples of recent outbreaks of** *E. coli* '**food poisoning**'

Canadian water and other authorities in the small town of Walkerton, Ontario, were sued for $C300m (£135m) after Canada's worst incident of contamination of water by *E. coli*, in which 2000 of the town's 5000 residents became ill and 14 died.

From a news report: Spurgeon D 2000 Canadians launch class action over *E coli* outbreak, BMJ, 321:11

Britain's worst outbreak of food poisoning from *E. coli* occurred in the Scottish town of Wishaw in 1996 and was initially linked to cold and cooked meat products supplied by a local butcher to dozens of outlets in the surrounding area. It resulted in five deaths and left 280 people ill. The deaths all occurred in elderly people who shared a meal at a church. All had eaten a steak pie, later found to contain *E. coli* in the gravy. Some children also became seriously ill and required kidney dialysis.

From a news report in: Christie B 1996 *E. Coli* kills five people in Scotland. BMJ 313:1424

Gastrointestinal infections

- Gastrointestinal infections, usually resulting in diarrhoea with or without vomiting, are very common but most cases are minor and do not need medical treatment.

- They are caused by bacteria and viruses contaminating food and are passed on through the faeces of infected persons usually by them in turn contaminating food then eaten by other people.

- Good food hygiene, particularly hand-washing and thorough cooking, would prevent many infections from spreading.

- Infected persons should not handle food intended for others.

- Occasional serious illness and even death does result from some infections, particularly in children and the elderly.

Infections and infestations of the skin

Infections of the skin are amongst the commonest of diseases. Most people will have experienced one or other of these at some time. Skin infections are broadly of three types:

- fungal
- viral
- bacterial.

This section deals only with some common examples, and we also exclude generalised rashes due to the specific infectious fevers of childhood, such as measles and chickenpox.

Fungal infections

The common fungal infections used to be called 'ringworm' because the rash can look worm shaped (Fig. 1), but there is no connection with worms of any kind. Fungi tend to grow particularly in moist, warm conditions, and infections can be passed from person to person through common facilitites such as showers and swimming baths. 'Athlete's foot' is the commonest form but fungi can also affect the scalp, any part of the body, but particularly around the genital area and the nails.

Another separate kind of fungal infection is 'thrush' or candidiasis. It is again common in warm moist areas such as the skinfolds, genital area and vagina itself, although it can affect virtually any part of the body. Obesity, diabetes and antibiotic use are thought to encourage thrush to develop. Vulvo-vaginal thrush will usually cause a whiteish vaginal discharge in addition to the skin inflammation.

Most of these infections are relatively harmless and susceptible to treatment.

Viral infections

The commonest skin infection is undoubtedly the verruca or common wart. Warts are due to human papilloma virus (HPV). They most commonly affect the hands (Fig. 2) or the soles of the feet but they can also occur on the penis or female genital area. Molluscum contagiosum is a less common condition, caused by a different virus, but generally similar in its effects (Fig. 3) and equally harmless. Our third and final example is cold sores (Fig. 4) which are due to a virus called herpes simplex. Cold sores arise because the virus lies dormant in the skin and flares up from time to time. They are not serious but can be difficult to eradicate. The herpes virus can also affect the genital areas and be transmitted by sexual intercourse.

Shingles (Fig. 5) is caused when the chickenpox virus (herpes zoster, quite a different virus from herpes simplex) is re-activated, usually in adulthood or old age, in someone who has already had chickenpox as a child. The virus lies dormant in the nervous system of the body and, when reactivated, spreads down a nerve to cause a blistery rash on the area of skin supplied by that nerve (see the dermatome chart on page 78).

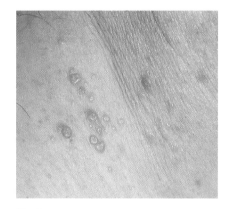

Fig. 3 **Molluscum contagiosum on the neck.** Source: Gawkrodger (2002).

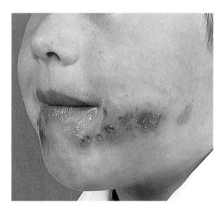

Fig. 4 Cold sores on the face of a child. Source: Gawkrodger (2002).

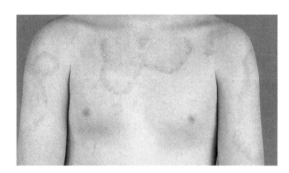

Fig. 1 **Tinea corporis ('ringworm'), showing a ring pattern.** Source: Wilkinson and Shaw (1998).

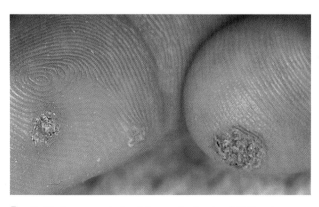

Fig. 2 **Viral warts** on the hand. Source: Gawkrodger (2002).

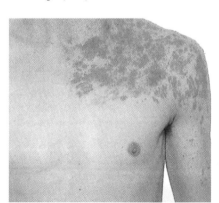

Fig. 5 **Herpes zoster (shingles)** in early stages, showing a characteristic 'band' distribution, here affecting left dermatomes C4 and C5. Source: Forbes and Jackson (1997).

Case history

A 25-year-old single mother brings her 6-week old baby to see the doctor with oral thrush. The baby is already sucking on a soother. The doctor notices that the 2-year old sister has peri-oral impetigo. Mother then asks for 'something' for her 6-year old daughter who is at home with an itchy rash. Looking at her case reports you discover that she has been prescribed treatment for scabies on a number of occasions over the past 12 months. You consider that the hygiene of this vulnerable family is poor. How are you going to help this family and what pharmacological agents will you use, and which members of the primary care team will you involve in the continuing care of this family?

Don't read this until you have come to some conclusions of your own!
The main underlying problem here is an educational one and it needs a coordinated approach from the primary health care team. Nowadays, a problem of this kind might present directly to the nurse prescriber in the UK and the doctor might not be involved. Generally, however, the response would come from the general practitioner and a health visitor or public health nurse. It would be important for one or other practitioner, probably the health visitor, to visit the family home to assess home conditions and to tailor the educational approach to this. It is unlikely that a single session would be enough to educate the mother properly and, in any case, further visits would be needed to check that education is being effective and hygiene is improving. It would be essential to take a friendly and supportive approach, rather than being judgemental, and to point out what would be the direct benefits to the family. For example, they would be healthier and the mother in the end would save time spent in looking after the children. Scabies can be treated with anti-scabetic lotions which are applied all over the body. All the family must be treated at the same time and there are other measures that need to be taken to ensure that the scabies mite does not survive the treatments and re-occur. The health visitor or other health worker would be best to supervise the treatment more closely than usual. Antibiotics could be prescribed for the impetigo and treatment given for the baby's oral thrush but, for example, it would be important to take other measures to prevent recurrence of infection, such as getting rid of the baby's soother (which may be carrying infection) or, at least, sterilising it with suitable chemicals from time to time.

Infestations

The common infestations of the skin are fleas, lice and scabies. These infestations are not necessarily connected with poor body hygiene and commonly occur in individuals who pride themselves on their cleanliness. There has to be some element of contact with another individual who has the infestation, therefore these infestations are more common where accommodation (particularly sleeping accommodation) is widely shared, for example in student accommodation, military barracks and oil rigs. Fleas are most commonly caught from pets and these animal fleas usually cause only a few bites on humans, as they prefer the animal host. Human fleas are more persistent but fortunately less common. Head lice are virtually epidemic in most school age children in the UK but other manifestations, e.g. pubic and body infestation are relatively rare. Although invariably precipitating much disgust in the parents (who are often from well-to-do homes) head lice are really quite benign and cause little real trouble, but can be quite difficult to eradicate. Scabies spreads within families more than within institutions, and seems to require quite close contact. In order of size, lice are probably the largest of the three and are easily seen, although the white eggs or 'nits' are much smaller. Lice are slow moving but fleas, which are rather smaller, can jump quite quickly. Scabies is caused by a mite which is virtually invisible to human sight. The mite burrows into the skin and, although this may be visible, it is usually the scratch marks caused by the intense itching reaction which are seen. A generalised itch over the whole body can be produced by a single mite.

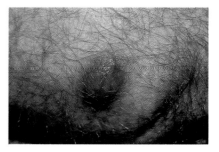

Fig. 6 **Boil or furuncle.** Source: White (1997).

Although very uncommon in the UK, insects can transmit infections via their bites, as where the mosquito passes on malaria, or where ticks from deer and other animals can transmit Lyme disease. Finally, there are other kinds of parasite, particularly protozoa, which commonly cause skin disease in tropical countries, but are not dealt with here.

Bacterial infections

There are a number of general infections affecting the body as a whole which also produce skin rashes. Examples include scarlet fever, where a generalised skin rash is produced in association with streptococcal infection of the throat. Also, bacteria (and fungi) can *secondarily* infect existing skin diseases, such as eczema. However, we deal particularly here with *primary* infections of the skin. Most readers will know of the common types, such as boils (folliculitis) and impetigo (Figs 6 and 7). These are usually caused by bacteria called *Staphylococci* or, less frequently, *Streptococci*, both of which can be treated with antibiotics. Against the need for antibotic treatment has to be set the dangers of producing antibiotic resistance, particularly in *staphylococci*.

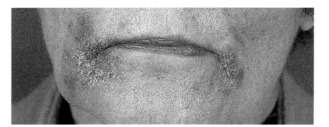

Fig. 7 **Impetigo.** Source: Gawkrodger (2002).

Infections and infestations of the skin

- Skin infections are very common and are usually contracted from other people who have the infection.
- Fungi, viruses and bacteria are the usual causes.
- Fungal infections commonly cause 'athlete's foot' and 'thrush'.
- Viral infections are commonly responsible for warts and 'cold sores'.
- Bacteria commonly cause boils and impetigo.
- Usually all of these infections can be easily treated.

Chronic skin disease

About 10% of GP consultations are for skin diseases (Table 1). This section does not deal with skin infections, including viral warts and fungal infections, which altogether account for about a third of consultations for skin disease. (see 'Infections of the Skin' pp 54–55)

Although the common chronic skin diseases can affect all age groups, atopic eczema is most common in infants, acne in adolescents and psoriasis in young adulthood.

There is a constitutional element in all three conditions that makes curative treatment difficult to obtain. In atopic eczema, which affects about 5 per 100 infants, there is usually a family history of atopy (an inherited tendency to develop allergies). In acne, the sebaceous glands of the hair follicles are hyperresponsive to androgen hormones, and in psoriasis, there is a strong hereditary influence associated with the HLA antigens CW6, B13 and B17.

Table 1 **Incidence of skin disease**

Rates of consultation (general practice) per 1000/year

All skin diseases	120.0
Dermatitis and eczema	45.6
Virus warts	14.3
Rash	13.3
Acne	9.6
Urticaria	8.6
Psoriasis	4.6
Chronic ulcer	2.4
Malignant neoplasms	0.8
Some comparisons	
Back pain	32.8
Osteoarthritis	23.5
Diseases of stomach	19.7
Irritable bowel	18.4
Rheumatoid arthritis	5.6

Source: Souhami and Moxham (1997)

Atopic eczema
'Eczema' is a relatively non-specific term for non-infective inflammation of the skin. There are other kinds of eczema (e.g. contact dermatitis), which will not be dealt with here.

Atopic eczema usually starts in the first year of life, often within the first few months. The appearance of the rash varies: acute lesions are different from chronic ones, the pattern also varying with age. Babies usually have an itchy rash on the face (Fig. 1), whereas after about 18 months of age the pattern tends to change to flexural eczema, affecting the backs of the

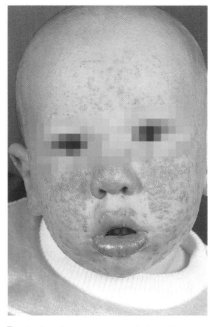

Fig. 1 **Atopic eczema in an infant.** Source: Gawkrodger (2002).

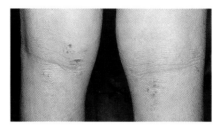

Fig. 2 **Atopic eczema involving the popliteal fossa in a child.** Source: Gawkrodger (2002).

elbows and knees and the folds of the neck, wrists and ankles (Fig. 2).

The outcome is generally good because the condition usually resolves by about 15 years of age without any damage to the skin. Some adults may continue to have contact dermatitis, usually of the hands, exacerbated by irritant chemicals or stress. There is no 'cure', but many treatments can make the condition much more tolerable and prevent skin damage caused by scratching.

Psoriasis
It is thought that factors such as infection, drugs (for example lithium and anti-malarials) and stress cause psoriasis to occur in genetically predisposed individuals. There is a variety of different appearances, plaque and flexural psoriasis (Figs 3 and 4) being the common chronic forms. The scalp and nails are often affected. Guttate psoriasis (Fig. 5) is the

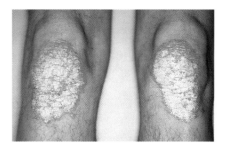

Fig. 3 **Typical scaly plaques of psoriasis on the knees.** Source: Gawkrodger (2002).

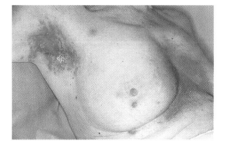

Fig. 4 **Smooth, non-keratotic involvement in flexural psoriasis.** Source: Gawkrodger (2002).

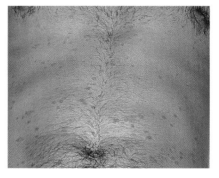

Fig. 5 **The drop-like lesions of guttate psoriasis.** Source: Gawkrodger (2002).

common acute form; it often occurs after streptococcal throat infections in younger people. Unlike the other, more chronic forms, it frequently resolves completely and so is important to recognise.

Psoriasis can be serious. There is a severe generalised form of pustular psoriasis that is fortunately rare, but about 5% of psoriasis sufferers (like the late playwright, Denis Potter), develop joint disease which can be very disabling. In addition the very powerful treatments that may be necessary in severe forms of psoriasis (for example methotrexate) can themselves have life-threatening effects.

Acne vulgaris
Acne usually starts at about 12 years of age and peaks at about 18 years in

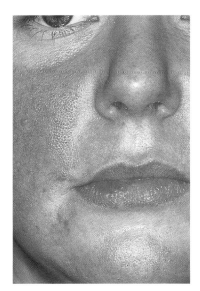

Fig. 6 **Acne rosacea.** Source: Wilkinson and Shaw (1999).

both sexes, affecting the areas of the body (face, shoulders, back and upper chest) where the sebaceous oily glands are most plentiful.

Factors involved in acne include:

- increased sebum secretion
- pilosebaceous duct hyperkeratosis
- infection with *Propionibacterium acnes*
- the release of inflammatory mediators.

The typical acne 'spot' is a comedone, either 'open' (a 'blackhead', which is a dilated pore with a plug of keratin stained by the pigment melanin) or 'closed' (a 'whitehead' with a cream-coloured top). In severe forms, these become much larger cysts and abcesses that then leave disfiguring permanent scars. Most patients improve by their late 20s, but a few still have acne into middle age.

Acne rosacea

Acne rosacea is a chronic inflammation of the nose and cheeks (or 'butterfly' distribution) that usually starts in middle age (Fig. 6). The cause is unknown but it may respond to treatments similar to those used for acne vulgaris.

Leg ulcers

Although ulcers may occur in other parts of the body, particularly due to tropical disease which we do not deal with here, the commonest kind of skin ulcer in the western world is very much the gravitational ulcer of the lower leg (Fig. 7), due simply to the effect of swelling of the legs with accumulated fluid, as a result of

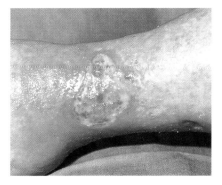

Fig. 7 **Gravitational ulcer of the lower leg.** Source: Gawkrodger (2002).

varicose veins and the pressure of gravity. These ulcers tend to occur in elderly patients and are difficult to heal, and so are best prevented by treatment of the underlying varicose veins before ulceration occurs. More rarely, if the arteries supplying blood to the leg are severely narrowed, the blood supply may be so poor that an ischaemic ulcer develops. This is even more serious and usually needs vascular surgery.

Melanoma

Melanomas are by far the commonest kind of skin cancer. Practically everyone has pigmented lesions ('moles') on the skin which are generally harmless but sometimes, because of exposure to too much sunlight, these moles become malignant cancers. This is more likely to happen in fair skinned people who are exposed to high levels of sunlight so that it is, for example, particularly common in fair skinned Australians. If a mole changes in colour or size, or particularly if it bleeds, it is important to get it checked. Melanomas (Fig. 8) can spread very rapidly throughout the body, often affect young people, and can be fatal if not treated quickly. Basal cell carcinomas (which may ulcerate as 'Rodent ulcers') are the other common type of skin cancer (Fig. 9). They are

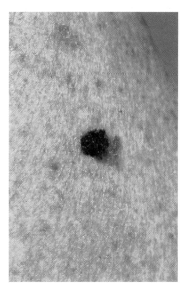

Fig. 8 **Malignant melanoma.** Source: Wilkinson and Shaw (1999).

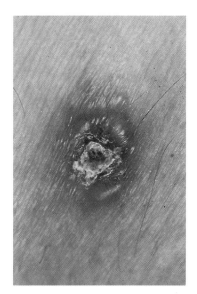

Fig. 9 **Basal cell carcinoma** with characteristic rolled, pearly border. Source: Wilkinson and Shaw (1999).

also caused by too much ultraviolet light exposure but are not pigmented, tend to occur in elderly or middle aged people, particularly on the face, and are generally not nearly as dangerous as melanoma.

Chronic skin disease

- About 10% of all GP consultations are for skin diseases.

- This section deals mainly with chronic (long term) skin disease – eczema, psoriasis and acne.

- There is a constitutional element in all three that makes it difficult to find curative treatments.

- Although the effects are mainly confined to the skin, psoriasis occasionally effects joints and other parts of the body, with potentially lethal effects.

- Each disease – eczema, psoriasis and acne – presents in different ways according to age and other factors, so that there is no one appearance universally typical of each disease.

Obstructive airways disease: asthma and chronic bronchitis

About 20% of general practice consultations are for respiratory symptoms, and, although well over half of these are for upper respiratory tract symptoms (see pp. 50–51), more than a quarter (about 1 in every 20 consultations, or 2 per day for the average GP) are for lower respiratory tract complaints, predominantly obstructive airways disease (OAD) (Fig. 1).

Although they are quite different diseases, we will consider chronic bronchitis and asthma together under the heading 'OAD' because they both result in obstruction to expiration. The symptoms and signs are therefore similar, and the two disorders may co-exist and be difficult to distinguish clinically.

Chronic bronchitis

The main cause of chronic bronchitis is tobacco-smoking, although atmospheric pollution is an additional factor. Increased airways resistance is caused by excess mucus secretion from an enlargement of the bronchial mucus glands and from a thickening of the bronchial wall. Some of these changes may initially be reversible on the cessation of smoking, but more permanent damage to the elastic tissue of the lungs (emphysema) is caused by a release of proteolytic enzymes and by the impairment of the natural protease inhibiting enzyme, alpha-1-antitrypsin.

Hereditary alpha-1-antitrypsin deficiency occurs in 1: 5000 individuals and may accelerate the development of emphysema in those affected individuals who smoke tobacco. These patients may develop chronic bronchitis early in life (before the age of 40). Chronic bronchitis is usually not obvious until age 50 or over because the initial symptom (increased sputum production) is trivial. Once significant symptoms (breathlessness on exercise) start to occur, the disease is usually irreversible, progressing in a proportion of patients to death from respiratory failure.

Bronchial asthma

On the other hand, permanent lung damage is unusual in bronchial asthma, an episodic, rather than chronic, disorder in which the the bronchi (which can be thought of as a tube of smooth muscle) 'clamp down' because of hypersensitivity to various trigger factors (Table 1). Industrial agents such as cotton dust (leading to byssinosis), wood dust and soldering flux may also cause occupational asthma. Asthma is therefore an essentially reversible disorder, although secondary factors (Fig. 2) may prolong an attack. At least 50% of

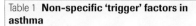

Table 1 **Non-specific 'trigger' factors in asthma**
■ Upper respiratory tract infection
■ Exercise
■ Cold air
■ Laughter
■ Irritants: smoke, paint and chemical fumes
■ Drugs, e.g. beta-blockers
■ Industrial causes

asthmatics have inherited an allergic tendency (atopy) as shown by a family history of this or other kinds of allergic reaction (e.g. allergic rhinitis, or 'hayfever', and eczema). Plant pollens (tree pollens in the spring and grass pollens in summer) and house dust mite (all year round) are the most common allergens.

Unlike chronic bronchitis, asthma occurs in all age groups. The peak in childhood is largely caused by allergy (*extrinsic* asthma) whereas late-onset asthma, often in middle age, is usually *intrinsic*, with no obvious allergic cause (although a family history of asthma is often present) (Table 2). Asthmatic attacks cease altogether by young adulthood in about 50% of young sufferers, and they are also often completely 'normal' between attacks. Late-onset asthma is more insidious, chronic and difficult to treat.

Although fundamentally a temporary phenomenon, asthma can be an exceedingly dangerous disease. Every year, 2000 asthmatics die in the UK, most within 2 hours of onset of an acute attack. Three out of four of these deaths are thought to be potentially preventable.

Respiratory failure

In both chronic bronchitis and asthma, death can occur from respiratory failure. Airways obstruction progressively limits oxygen entry to the lung tissue. There is normally a considerable tolerance to a variation in oxygen supply, but, at a critical point (Fig. 3) a further reduction in oxygen entry causes a drastically disproportionate fall in oxygen carriage by the blood (percentage saturation of haemoglobin), with rapidly increasing danger to life itself. Central cyanosis (cyanosis in normally warm areas of the body, such as the tongue, rather than in peripheral areas like the lips or

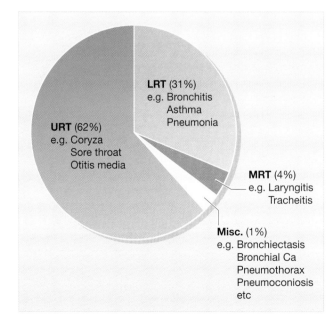

Fig. 1 **Consultations for respiratory disease (approximately one fifth of all consultations).**
URT: upper respiratory tract; LRT: lower respiratory tract: MRT: middle respiratory tract

LRT (31%)
e.g. Bronchitis
Asthma
Pneumonia

URT (62%)
e.g. Coryza
Sore throat
Otitis media

MRT (4%)
e.g. Laryngitis
Tracheitis

Misc. (1%)
e.g. Bronchiectasis
Bronchial Ca
Pneumothorax
Pneumoconiosis
etc

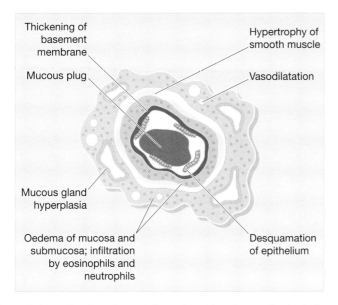

Fig. 2 **The pathology of asthma.** Intense inflammation, with oedema and intraluminal mucous plugs, is the striking pathology of asthma. Source: Souhami and Moxham (1994)

Table 3 **Danger signs in asthma – admission to hospital is needed**

- Difficulty speaking because of breathlessness
- Use of the accessory muscles of respiration
- A rapid heart rate
- A peak flow rate of less than 100 L/min
- 'Pulsus paradoxus' – a pulse pressure that is reduced during inspiration (usually detected with a sphygmomanometer)
- Greatly reduced air entry or even a 'silent' chest on auscultation
- Any degree of central cyanosis

Other warning features

- Past medical history of hospital treatment for a severe attack
- Extremes of age
- A serious complication in a previous attack
- Great distress or anxiety
- Poor social circumstances

Table 2 **The classification of extrinsic and intrinsic asthma**

Extrinsic	Intrinsic
History of allergy (e.g. hay-fever and eczema)	No allergic history
Skin tests positive	Skin tests negative
Early onset	Late onset
Family history of atopy	Family history of asthma only
Intermittent attacks, often seasonal	Persisting asthma, perennial
Elevated IgE level	Normal IgE level
Marked blood and sputum eosinophilia	Variable eosinophilia
Not aspirin sensitive, occasional polyps	Aspirin sensitive, nasal polyps
Good response to beta-agonists	Variable response to beta-agonists
Good response to Sodium cromoglicate	Poor response to sodium cromoglicate

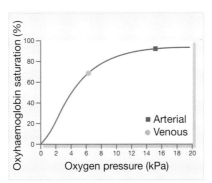

Fig. 3 **Oxygen dissociation curve.** In normal subjects, a large fall in arterial oxygen tension causes a small reduction in oxyhaemoglobin saturation (and oxygen carriage). In the hypoxic patient (for example, with a PaO_2 of 6 kPa), a small fall in oxygen tension causes marked desaturation.

hands) indicates that the oxygen saturation of the blood is less than 85% (usually much less if it can be easily detected).

In the early stages of an asthma attack, rapid breathing washes carbon dioxide out of the lungs more quickly than usual, but in a severe attack this is reversed. Carbon dioxide retention causes acidosis of the blood, which progressively inactivates the brain centres that stimulate breathing.

Carbon dioxide retention is, however, much more commonly a feature of chronic bronchitis. Giving a high level of oxygen 'fools' the brain into thinking that even less respiratory effort is required, despite the high carbon dioxide levels, and results in a further dangerous depression of breathing. This is why only low-concentration (24 or 28%) oxgen is used when carbon dioxide retention is suspected.

Danger signs
These, fundamentally, indicate a dangerously low oxygen saturation caused by respiratory depression with or without carbon dioxide retention. They indicate, particularly in asthmatics, one of the most urgent and dangerous emergencies in medicine (Table 3).

Routine management
Although constant alertness to it is vital, dangerous episodes are fortunately, relatively rare, most primary health care being focused on the alleviation of symptoms and proactive management (tertiary prevention) to try to limit the future effect of these diseases. The main treatment for asthma is inhaled medication, which can be divided into two main types:

- *bronchodilators*, which have a rapid action in relieving spasm of the bronchial muscle
- *preventive treatments*, mainly inhaled steroids, which are used in very small doses to suppress the heightened sensitivity of the bronchial mucus membrane that occurs in asthma, so that it does not then react to various allergens and irritants.

Box 1 Good care of obstructive airways disease

Pneumococcal vaccination
Annual 'flu vaccine'
Beta agonist e.g. salbutamol
Nicotine replacement therapy for smokers
Rotate antibiotics
Chest physiotherapy

Obstructive airways disease

- Obstructive airways disease, predominantly caused by chronic bronchitis and/or asthma accounts for about 5% of GP consultations.
- Chronic bronchitis is caused by cigarette smoking and leads to permanent lung damage with severe disability and early death in many individuals.
- Asthma is essentially a reversible episodic disorder, with little or no lasting lung damage, at least in younger age groups.
- However, life-threatening respiratory failure may occur in both diseases and can be especially sudden and dangerous in asthma.

Diabetes mellitus I

Glucose is a simple sugar that is essential for brain and muscle activity. The hormone insulin is necessary to use glucose as energy, and if there is a shortage of insulin, or if it does not function properly, glucose will accumulate and diabetes develop.

There are two main types of diabetes:

- *Insulin-dependent diabetes (IDDM)* occurs when there is a severe lack of insulin as a result of the destruction of most, or all, of the insulin-producing islet cells in the pancreas. This type usually occurs before the age of 40 years and develops rapidly.
- *Non-insulin-dependent diabetes (NIDDM)* was previously known as type 2 diabetes. Here, the body may still be producing some insulin, but in an inadequate amount, alternatively, if insulin is being produced, it is not available to work properly. The glucose level can be reduced by improved diet or tablets, although insulin injections may sometimes be needed. NIDDM usually occurs over the age of 40 and is of gradual onset.

Causes

In IDDM, the destruction of the insulin-producing islet cells is believed to be caused by an autoimmune process that may well be triggered off in susceptible individuals by unidentified viruses and chemicals. Susceptibility may be genetically determined. In NIDDM, insulin is still produced but in an insufficient quantity, or else its functioning is impaired. Defects in the islet cells are thought to be responsible for insulin deficiency, but insulin resistance in muscles and other tissues is evident in nearly all individuals with NIDDM. The condition tends to run in families, and it is likely that several genes are involved. Contributory factors include increasing age, obesity and a sedentary life-style.

How common is diabetes?

The great majority of people with diabetes are non-insulin dependent, this accounting for between 75% and 90% of cases of the condition. In the Poole Diabetes Study of newly diagnosed type 2 diabetics (1996–98) the crude incidence was 2/1000 patients. The incidence was much

Table 1 **The prevalence of diabetes (known and previously undiagnosed) in people of Asian and European origin**

Age (years)	Prevalence: Men (%)		Prevalence: Women (%)	
	Asian	European	Asian	European
20–39	2.5	0.5	1.5	0.5
40–59	12.5	3.5	9.5	6.0
60–79	25.5	6.5	20.0	8.0

higher in older men (6.5/1000) than in women of equivalent age. There is a large ethnic difference in the prevalence of diabetes, the figure in those of Asian and Afro-Caribbean origin being higher than seen in Europeans (Table 1).

Undiagnosed diabetes

This can only be estimated by screening population samples, but surveys indicate that the ratio of undiagnosed to diagnosed diabetes may be as high as 1:1.

Early diagnosis

All patients at risk should be screened frequently as early diagnosis and immediate treatment is important. Patients at risk of type 2 diabetes are those over 55 years, obese, hyperlipidaemic, with a family history of diabetes and skin or urine infections.

Box 1

Diabetes is confirmed if:
- Random or two hour post prandial glucose greater than 11 mmol/L
- Fasting glucose greater than 7 mmol/L

Diabetes is excluded if:
- Random glucose is less than 5.5 mmol/L
- Two hour post prandial glucose is less than 7.8 mmol/L
- Fasting glucose is less than 6 mmol/L

Impaired glucose tolerance:
- Two hour post prandial glucose 7.8–11 mmol/L

Risk factor modification

Modifying lifestyle is an important area in the management of diabetes. Patients should be advised regarding the balance of their diet, alcohol intake and weight reduction. Regular aerobic exercise has an important effect on the

metabolism of glucose and the promotion of smoking cessation in at risk patients is important.

Achieving glycaemic control

HbAlc reflects glycaemic controls over the previous 6 weeks and is now used for the basis of treatment decisions. Ideally it should be measured every 6 months in diabetic patients. In patients who are obese an HbA_{1c} less than 6.5% is a difficult but worthwhile target. In those patients who are not obese a target of less than 7.5% is sufficient. There may be a risk of hypoglycaemic episodes and patients need advice on managing such episodes. As a rule of thumb, every 1% reduction in HbA_{1c} can reduce the risk of myocardial infarction or stroke by approximately 15% and further reduces the risk of peripheral vascular disease by 40%.

Patients can now be taught to monitor their blood at home which can be done daily and recorded at fasting, pre-prandial and bed times. Urine testing is less invasive and is acceptable if the blood results are consistently negative and HbA_{1c} targets are met.

Hypertension

Hypertension is extremely common in type 2 diabetes with 40% of type 2 diabetics having hypertension at the age of 45 and 60% having hypertension at the age of 75. Evidence indicates that tight blood pressure control, aiming for less than 130/85 is more important than glycaemic control in reducing morbidity and mortality. Weight reduction, salt reduction and exercise are the first line treatment in hypertension and this is even more important in diabetics.

Lipids

Before considering medication for the control of hyperlipidemia, glycaemic control should be sought through lifestyle and in particular dietary modification. As in non-diabetics, total cholesterol should be less than 5 mmol/L, total HDL less than 4 mmol/L, LDL cholesterol less than 3 mmol/L. The total cholesterol: HDL ratio should be less than 5. Stains are now the medication of choice, except where triglycerides are markedly elevated and a fibrate is maybe more appropriate.

Complications

Microvascular

Microvascular complications (caused by to damage to the small blood vessels) include:

- retinopathy
- nephropathy
- neuropathy.

Retinopathy. In the European multi-centre study of 3250 people with IDDM, background retinopathy was found in 36% and proliferative retinopathy in 10% of cases. The prevalence is related to the duration of diabetes, but as many as 18% of people with NIDDM have diabetic retinopathy at the time of diagnosis. Diabetes is the single most common cause of blindness among adults in the 16–64-year-age group. These figures show a steady decline compared with those for previous years, this being related to the better monitoring and treatment of diabetes. It is recommended that patients with diabetes undergo fundoscopy on an annual basis (Fig. 1).

Nephropathy. Like retinopathy, nephropathy is declining, especially in IDDM, but it still develops in 20–25% of people with diabetes. It used to be thought that nephropathy occured in a smaller proportion of people with NIDDM, but studies from Denmark

and the USA indicate that the cumulative incidence of nephropathy in NIDDM is 20–25%, as in IDDM.

Nephropathy takes 10–15 years to develop and leads to a progressively rising level of albumin in the urine. No other symptoms exist at this stage, but as kidney function declines, uraemic symptoms, such as tiredness, nausea, shortness of breath and oedema of the limbs, appear. The progression of nephropathy can be delayed by restricting dietary protein and by careful blood pressure control. Angiotensin-converting enzyme inhibitors have a significant benefit that is only in part the result of their effect on blood pressure.

The treatment of choice for end-stage renal failure is kidney transplantation. Over the past few years, the results with renal transplantation in diabetics have improved, now being comparable to those seen in non-diabetic patients. The early detection of nephropathy allows intervention before the patient progresses to established nephropathy. An annual urine check for albumin is advised by the British Diabetic Association.

Neuropathy. Two main types of neuropathy occur in association with diabetes:

1 *sensorimotor peripheral neuropathy*, which impairs touch, heat and pain sensation
2 *autonomic neuropathy*, which impairs involuntary control of the heart and blood vessels.

It has been estimated that the prevalence of neuropathy is just over 16% in people with diabetes, compared with 3% in the non-diabetic population. The prevalence of

autonomic neuropathy seems to be higher, at 40%, but this is usually asymptomatic. Symptoms of sensory neuropathy include tingling, burning, cramps, and pain and numbness in a glove or stocking distribution. Autonomic neuropathy can cause poor control of the blood pressure, leading to postural hypotension, bladder and bowel emptying problems and disturbances of sweating. Erectile impotence may affect 50% of male diabetics.

Macrovascular and other complications

Macrovascular complications (arising from damage to the larger arteries) include:

- *ischaemic or coronary heart disease* affecting the blood supply to the heart, manifesting as angina and myocardial infarction
- *cerebrovascular disease*, affecting the blood vessels in the brain and leading to strokes
- *peripheral vascular disease*, affecting the blood supply to the legs and causing intermittent claudication and gangrene if severe.

Other complications may affect the feet, the skin, the joints and tendons, the gastrointestinal tract and sexual function.

Cardiovascular disease. Cardiovascular disease is a major cause of chronic ill-health in the population in general, and in those with diabetes there is a 2–3-fold increase in coronary heart disease in men and a 4–5-fold, increased risk in pre-menopausal women. The risk of stroke is also increased 2–3-fold, and peripheral vascular disease greatly increases the risk of intermittent claudication, gangrene and amputation.

The major risk factors for cardiovascular disease in the population in general – hypertension, a raised cholesterol level, smoking, obesity and physical inactivity – also apply to people with diabetes, but diabetes appears to be an additional risk factor.

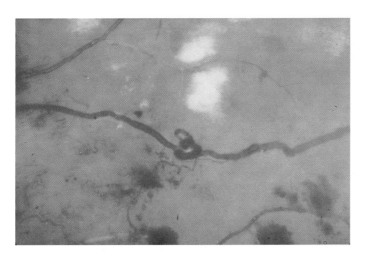

Fig. 1 **Retinopathy.** Source: Forbes and Jackson (1991).

Diabetes mellitus II

The diabetic foot

Diabetics are prone to ulceration and gangrene of the lower limb, which greatly increases the risk of amputation (Fig. 1). The prevalence of foot ulceration was found to be 7.4% in people with diabetes compared with 2.5% in a non-diabetic comparison group. The main factors responsible for foot problems in diabetes are neuropathy and ischaemia, often in combination with infection as a provoking and complicating factor.

Ulcers can develop as the result of mechanical trauma from callus formation, ill-fitting shoes or burns from hot water bottles. Because of neuropathy, these may have progressed to an advanced stage before they are felt or noticed. An impaired blood supply from peripheral vascular disease impairs healing, and sepsis can spread rapidly, destroying bone and soft tissues.

Foot problems can be prevented by alerting the patient to the importance of good footcare and good chiropody; a foot clinic at King's College Hospital, London, reduced the number of amputations occurring from 12 to five per annum.

Diabetes and pregnancy

Although the perinatal mortality rate (including the number of stillbirths and neonatal deaths) has fallen dramatically over the past 50 years, it is still higher for diabetic women, at 56 per 1000 births, than for the general population (14 per 1000 births). Major congenital malformations are responsible for about one third of these deaths, the overall incidence of congenital malformation in diabetic being 7%.

The babies of mothers with diabetes tend to be larger at birth and to have an increased risk of respiratory distress syndrome and hypoglycaemia.

Maternal mortality is thought to be higher in diabetic than non-diabetic women.

Gestational diabetes

A number of women are found to have diabetes during pregnancy. This may disappear for a few years after the pregnancy, but as many as 50% of women with gestational diabetes subsequently develop non-insulin dependent diabetes (NIDDM). The impact of gestational diabetes on the pregnancy is similar to that of established diabetes but with fewer and less severe complications.

Mortality

Mortality statistics are notoriously unreliable, and in diabetes the cause of death may be attributed to a complication rather than to the diabetes itself. Indeed, in older patients, the condition may not even be mentioned on the death certificate. A study by the British Diabetic Association demonstrated that, in under-50 age group, men with diabetes were 3.5 times and women 11 times more likely to die from cardiovascular disease than were a comparable group of non-diabetics. There has, however, been a fall in the level diabetes-related mortality over recent years.

The treatment of diabetes

Twenty per cent of those with diabetes are treated with diet alone, 50% with diet and tablets, and 30% with diet and insulin. The overall aim of treatment is to keep the blood glucose level as near normal as possible.

Diet

The general advice for people with diabetes is to eat a healthy diet, as recommended for everyone else. This means a diet that is low in sugar, low in fat and high in fibre. Special diabetic foods are expensive and confer no particular nutritional advantage.

Insulin

Most of the insulin now in use is produced by genetic engineering, but some animal insulin is still available for those who prefer it.

Commonly encountered insulin regimens (Table 1) are: a single daily dose of a long-acting insulin, used mostly in older people; four times daily injection with a short-acting insulin, injection being carried out before each of the three main meals for flexibility with good control; a combination of soluble with long-acting insulin, especially in the elderly or in NIDDM diabetics starting insulin.

The injections are given subcutaneously, the best sites being the abdomen, the outer thighs, the buttocks and the upper arms. Insulin pens containing pre-filled cartridges of insulin are increasingly being used for convenience, speed and ease of injection.

Commonly used oral hypoglycaemics

These are summarised in Box 1. The sulphonylureas work by stimulating the islet cells to produce more insulin. Metformin is thought to act by enhancing the uptake of glucose by individual cells; it is used in individuals who are obese and can be taken in combination with a sulphonylurea.

Acarbose has recently been introduced for the treatment of NIDDM. It inhibits the intestinal enzyme alpha-glucosidase, which digests complex sugars. By inhibiting this activity, the drug delays the increase in blood glucose level that occurs after a meal.

Why good control matters

Ten years ago, two large multi-centre studies were set up to investigate the degree to which the control of diabetes affected its complication rate. The Diabetes Control and Complications Trial was carried out in 29 centres in the USA and Canada, involving 1441

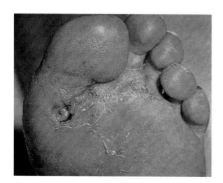

Fig. 1 **Diabetic foot.** Source: Forbes and Jackson (1991).

Table 1 **Classification of insulin preparations**		
	Appearance	**'Usual' pattern of use**
Short-acting	Clear	With meals, twice or more daily
Soluble (Actrapid)		Good control, provides flexibility, used in conjunction with long-term preparations
Long-acting	Cloudy	Once (or twice) daily, usually at night
Insulatard		
Combined/biphasic	Cloudy	Twice daily in a ratio of 30:70, 40:60 or 50:50.
(a combination of short and long acting)		Used especially for NIDDM or in the elderly

people with IDDM. It compared the effects of a conventional insulin treatment of one or two injections a day with an intensified regimen of two or more injections a day on the development of complications. The findings conclusively demonstrated that good blood glucose control reduced the risk of complications. There was:

- a 76% reduction in the risk of developing new instances of retinopathy
- a 54% reduction in the risk of progression of existing retinopathy
- a 39% reduction in the risk of developing microalbuminuria
- a 54% reduction in the risk of developing clinical albuminuria
- a 60% reduction in the risk of neuropathy
- a three-fold increase in the risk of severe hypoglycaemia with intensive therapy.

The UK Prospective Diabetes Study is currently being carried out on 5100 patients with NIDDM, treatment being randomised between diet alone, diet and oral hypoglycaemic drugs, and insulin injections; the results of the trial are still being awaited.

Family support

The diagnosis of diabetes involves psychological, social and work adjustments as well as education in self-care. Over 30% of new diabetics find themselves being unable to cope with the diagnosis and it is known that being unable to cope is a highly significant predictor of protracted psychological and compliance problems. A new diagnosis of diabetes mellitus involves the family as it considerably increases their risk of the illness. Modern diabetic control places a large emphasis on the patient in the control and maintenance of their chronic disease. Relatively little attention has been paid to the importance of the family for the adult diabetic. There is, however, evidence that non-supportive family behaviours are related to poor compliance and poor glucose control in adults. The relationship that patients have with their family members is a critical factor in improving their sense of well-being, which in turn leads to more effective self-management of diabetes. The DAWN study indicates that patients without family networks, especially those living alone, feel worse in themselves and do not manage the disease effectively.

Box 1 Commonly used oral hypoglycaemics

Sulphonylureas
- Glibenclamide (Daonil)
- Gliclazide (Diamicron)
- Glipizide (Glibinese)

Biguanide
- Metformin (Glucophage)

- *Acarbose* (Glucobay)

The organisation of care and general practice

Diabetes mellitus, particularly NIDDM, is commonly seen in general practice. It is easily diagnosed and easily missed, with a lifelong course that affects many parts of the body. Because of its multi-system effects, the organisation of care is extremely important; this should involve specialists, doctors, practice nurses, chiropodists and dieticians. The maintenance of a diagnostic register can greatly help the organisation and delivery of care within the practice. Many practices now have a diabetic clinic that can bring together many of the personnel involved in care for the patient while using specialist networks as appropriate.

Because of the dramatic presentation of IDDM, these patients have traditionally received more attention than those with NIDDM. It is, however, now becoming apparent that the complications of NIDDM are just as many and as serious as those of IDDM. Diabetes is a major and growing European health problem that causes prolonged ill-health and early death, threatening at least 10 million European citizens. In the face of such a major health problem, the organisation of care at both primary care and secondary care levels is of great importance. Opportunistic care of NIDDM does not work and regular reviews are needed, typically every 3 months extending to 6 or 12 months over time. Recall for non-attenders is necessary if medical care is to provide good control.

Table 2 **The diabetes consultation in general practice**

Topic for review	Initial review/refer	Regular review	Annual review
Background history			
Social history, lifestyle review		If problem	
Long-term or recent diabetes history	Consider referral		
Complications history/symptoms	Refer		
Other medical history/systems		✓	
Family history diabetes/arterial disease		✓	
Drug history/current drugs		✓	
Current skills/well-being			
Diabetes self-management			✓
Self-monitoring skills/results			✓
Vascular risk factors			
HbA₁c (glycated haemoglobin)	Refer if problem		
Lipid profile		If problem	
Blood pressure		If problem	
Smoking		If problem	
Urine albumin excretion (not if proteinuria)		If problem	
Examination/complications			
General examination	Initial review		✓
Weight/body mass index			✓
Foot examination		If problem	
Eye/vision examination		If problem	
Urine protein		If problem	
Serum creatinine		If problem	

Based on British College of General Practitioners Diabetes Task Force (2000)

Diabetes mellitus

- It is expected that 5–10% of the population will be affected by type 2 diabetes.
- Diabetes dramatically increases the risks of ischaemic heart disease and strokes
- Every 1% reduction in HbA₁c reduces risk of myocardial infarction or stroke by 15%.
- Microvascular disease affects the eye, kidney and peripheral nerves.
- Macrovascular disease affects the heart, brain and legs.
- Good control really matters.
- Being unable to cope is a predictor of psychological and compliance problems.

Hypertension

Blood pressure varies from person to person, and in the same individual under different circumstances: fear, pain and exercise can, for example, all cause a transient increase in blood pressure. Hypertension (raised blood pressure) occurs when the systolic and/or diastolic pressure, measured by a sphygmomanometer, is higher than 'normal' for that individual's age group (remembering that the average systolic blood pressure increases with age).

Both systolic and diastolic blood pressure have a normal or gaussian distribution within a community (Fig. 1). If a level of 140/90 mmHg were taken as the upper limit of normal, 10–15% of the whole population would be hypertensive. A more flexible definition of hypertension would therefore be 'the level of blood pressure above which investigation and treatment do more good than harm'. A GP with 2000 patients is likely to have up to 300 people with a blood pressure reading over 140/90 mmHg, but unless the practice has a screening policy, not all of these will have been identified.

The blood pressure should ideally be measured when the patient is at rest and relaxed (rather than right at the start of the consultation) and should be recorded on at least three separate occasions..

Morbidity and mortality increase significantly at higher levels of pressure as damage occurs to the heart, brain, kidneys and eyes

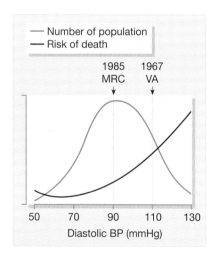

— Number of population
— Risk of death

1985 MRC   1967 VA

50   70   90   110   130
Diastolic BP (mmHg)

Fig. 1 Distribution of diastolic blood pressure (BP) in a Western population and risk of death. MRC: Medical Research Council; VA: Veterans Administration. (After Walker & Tan 2002).

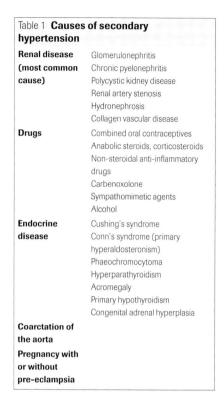

Table 1 **Causes of secondary hypertension**	
Renal disease (most common cause)	Glomerulonephritis
	Chronic pyelonephritis
	Polycystic kidney disease
	Renal artery stenosis
	Hydronephrosis
	Collagen vascular disease
Drugs	Combined oral contraceptives
	Anabolic steroids, corticosteroids
	Non-steroidal anti-inflammatory drugs
	Carbenoxolone
	Sympathomimetic agents
	Alcohol
Endocrine disease	Cushing's syndrome
	Conn's syndrome (primary hyperaldosteronism)
	Phaeochromocytoma
	Hyperparathyroidism
	Acromegaly
	Primary hypothyroidism
	Congenital adrenal hyperplasia
Coarctation of the aorta	
Pregnancy with or without pre-eclampsia	

(so-called 'target organ damage'). Hypertension is more common in females, certain ethnic groups (African-Americans and Japanese) and the inhabitants of countries with a high-salt diet.

There are two varieties of hypertension:

- *primary* or essential hypertension (95%), with no specific underlying cause
- *secondary hypertension* (5%), caused by a specific disease or abnormality (see Table 1).

Malignant hypertension occurs when there is a rapid increase in blood pressure, with progressive target organ damage and death within a few months in untreated cases. It is a medical emergency and requires immediate hospital admission.

Presentation

Hypertension produces no symptoms in the majority of patients, the diagnosis usually being made on routine examination when attending the doctor's surgery for an unrelated problem or a 'check-up'. Sixty per cent of newly diagnosed hypertensives have no symptoms, 20% have anxiety symptoms that may not be related to high blood pressure, and 20% have symptoms that may have been

associated with an awareness of hypertension (headache and nose bleeds) or with its complications:

- angina – coronary artery disease
- breathlessness – left ventricular failure
- intermittent claudication – peripheral vascular disease
- dizziness – carotid and cerebral arterial disease
- visual deterioration – retinal vascular disease
- polyuria, weight loss and anaemia – renal failure.

Most patients with hypertension show no abnormal physical signs apart from their raised blood pressure. A minority may show evidence of target organ damage, for example retinopathy, left ventricular hypertrophy or the after-effects of a stroke. Physical signs are more prominent in secondary hypertension, with, for example, reduced or absent femoral pulses in coarctation of the aorta, enlarged kidneys in polycystic disease or a plethoric moon face with Cushing's syndrome.

The consequences of target organ damage are:

- *heart*: coronary artery disease (angina and myocardial infarction)
- *brain*: cerebral arterial disease (transient ischaemic attacks and strokes)
- *kidneys*: chronic renal failure
- *eyes*: retinopathy (graded in severity from 1 to 4).

These will not, however, occur until much later in life. The purpose of identifying and treating hypertension at an asymptomatic stage is therefore to prevent these serious long-term consequences.

Diagnosis

The diagnosis of hypertension is based on a series of blood pressure measurements. In the absence of secondary hypertension or complications, the physical examination is usually unremarkable.

With essential hypertension, investigations can establish whether there has been any target organ damage and therefore provide guidance on prognosis:

- ECG – evidence of left ventricular hypertrophy and ischaemia

- CXR – evidence of cardiomegaly and heart failure
- urine analysis – evidence of proteinuria and haematuria
- plasma urea/creatinine level – showing renal failure.
- fasting lipids and glucose – risk factors

If secondary hypertension is suspected, special investigations are required; these may include the 24 hour urine catecholamines level to identify phaeochromocytoma, plasma renin and aldosterone levels for Conn's syndrome and a renal ultrasound for renal disease.

Management

The aims of treating hypertension are to reduce mortality and the risk of complications. Once established, treatment is usually lifelong. Management involves advice on life-style and risk factor control, and antihypertensive medication. Since most hypertensives are asymptomatic, the benefits of treatment have to be balanced against the possible side-effects and inconvenience (Table 2, Box 1).

General measures involve diet (weight reduction in the obese, reducing of heavy alcohol consumption and avoiding of adding salt at the table), regular non-competitive exercise, stopping smoking and reducing hyperlipidaemia.

The decision to institute drug treatment depends on the absolute level of blood pressure, the assessment of other risk factors, the presence of target organ damage and associated clinical conditions such as cardiovascular, cerebrovascular or renal disease (Table 3).

The main antihypertensive drug groups are:

- thiazide diuretics, for example bendrofluazide
- beta-blockers such as atenolol
- angiotensin-converting enzyme (ACE) inhibitors, for example captopril
- calcium-channel blockers, such as nifedipine
- angiotensin II receptor antagonists, for example losartan
- peripheral vasodilators, such as prazosin.

Organised care

Many general practices have now organised the identification and management of their hypertensive patients. Tagging notes so that all patients over 40 years old have their blood pressure checked every 5 years is good practice; this can be done opportunistically at ordinary consultations, or patients can be invited to attend for a check-up. Many practices have their own guidelines or protocols for diagnosis and management, and care is often shared between the doctor and practice nurse. Once the hypertension has been controlled, it is important to monitor the patient at regular intervals (every 3–6 months), some practices running 'mini-clinics' for hypertensives.

However, the rule of halves probably still exists: only half of all hypertensives are diagnosed, only half of these patients are treated, and the blood pressure is well controlled in only half of those receiving therapy.

Table 2 **Common side-effects of antihypertensive agents**	
Side-effect	**Associated drug(s)**
Postural hypotension	Diuretics, vasodilators
Gout	Diuretics
Impotence	Diuretics, beta-blockers
Cough	ACE inhibitors
Dyspnoea	Beta-blockers
Headache, flushing	Calcium-channel blockers
Lethargy	Beta-blockers

Box 1 **Number needed to treat**

In younger hypertensives (age 40–64), treatment for 833 patient–years is required to prevent one stroke, and there is no benefit in terms of the prevention of a coronary event. In older hypertensives (aged 65–75), treatment is required for 370 patient–years to prevent one stroke and for 417 patient–years to prevent one coronary event.

Table 3 **Stratification of absolute cardiovascular risk to quantify prognosis (WHO–ISH guidelines)**

		Blood pressure (mmHg)		
Other risk factors and disease history		Mild hypertension (Grade 1) SBP 140–159 or DBP 90–99	Moderate hypertension (Grade 2) SBP 160–179 or DBP 100–109	Severe hypertension (Grade 3) SBP ≤ 180 or DBP ≥ 110
I	No other risk factors	Low risk	Med. risk	High risk
II	1–2 risk factors	Med. risk	Med. risk	V. high risk
III	3 or more risk factors or TOD or diabetes	High risk	High risk	V. high risk
IV	ACC	V. high risk	V. high risk	V. high risk

SBP, systolic blood pressure; DBP, diastolic blood pressure; TOD, target organ damage; ACC, associated clinical conditions including clinical cardiovascular disease and renal disease.

Risk categories relate to risk of a cardiovascular event in the succeeding 10 years:
Low < 15%
Medium 15–20%
High 20–30%
Very high > 30%

Source: National Blood Pressure Advisory Committee 1999. Modified from: Guidelines Subcommittee of the WHO-ISH 1999

Hypertension

- Hypertension is common, affecting 1 in 7 adults.
- Ninety-five per cent of cases have no specific underlying cause.
- A GP with 2000 patents is likely to have up to 300 people with a blood pressure of over 140/90 mmHg.
- The risks associated with hypertension are of stroke, coronary artery disease, renal failure and premature death.
- Nearly all hypertensives can be managed in the community, but this requires good practice organisation and teamwork.
- The aims of management are to reduce mortality and the risks of complications.
- General measures involve weight reduction, the control of alcohol intake, a reduction of salt intake, regular exercise, stopping smoking and reducing hyperlipidaemia.
- Drugs used include diuretics, beta-blockers, ACE inhibitors, calcium-channel blockers, angiotensin II receptor antagonists and peripheral vasodilators.

Common mental health problems I

Mood disorders

The term 'mood disorders' applies to disorders in which the mood is either depressed or elated; they are classified into unipolar and bipolar disorders. Patients with a depressive disorder are broadly classified as unipolar depression, those with both depressive disorder and mania being broadly classified as having a bipolar disorder. Although the clinical features of unipolar depression and bipolar disorder are similar, important differences exist in the hereditary aspects. Between 10% and 20% bipolar disorders sufferers can have up to three episodes of depression before they develop a manic illness.

Depression

Depression is the most common mental health disorder seen in general practice, being present in about 10% of those who consult the GP. The lifetime risk of depression is 10% for men and 20% for women, although these figures are likely to be underestimates. Depression is an important cause of morbidity, disability and mortality.

Susceptibility to depression

Depression 'probably has no single cause but rather represents a personal response to a multitude of biological, psychological, social and cultural factors' (Wright 1999).

Gender. There is a significant difference in the consultation rate for depression between men and women, women in the 16–44-year age group consulting over three times as often than men. The ratio decreases slowly thereafter, but a greater proportion of women continue to consult for depression throughout all the age groups. This difference may represent a greater susceptibility of females to depression, or it may represent a greater likelihood of women consulting with depression. It is increasingly appreciated that men are less likely to consult for emotional and psychological difficulties, so some of the difference in consultation rate might be explained by a resistance to seeking medical help.

Biology. There is increasing interest in the genetics of psychological illnesses, with some evidence of a genetic basis to depression. A neurochemical hypothesis is that there is a reduced level of 5-hydroxytryptamine (5-HT) at the synapses, which is responsible for the condition. Noradrenaline (norepinephrine) has been similarly implicated, and the newer antidepressants (selective serotonin reuptake inhibitors) act by raising one central catecholamine level, particularly that of 5-HT and noradrenaline (morepinephrine).

Life events and stresses. Life events such as a new baby, divorce, job loss and moving house are known to provoke depressive episodes. Socio-economic deprivation is also an important risk factor for depression.

Family and personal support. The loss of a mother in childhood is an important risk factor for depression, as is caring for young children, especially those under the age of 5 years. The absence of a close confiding relationship and support from family and friends is also an important predictor of depression.

Grief. This is a normal and natural reaction to loss. It is difficult to put a time limit on a grief reaction, but fewer than 10% of those experiencing a recent loss develop a depressive illness, a prolonged grief reaction being symptomatic of depression.

Postnatal depression. This is depression following childbirth, to which are added feelings of inability to cope with the new baby and motherhood. Puerperal psychosis may rarely develop; in this, the mother's delusions may place the baby at risk of physical harm.

Menopause. This is associated with depression in many patients' and doctors' minds. The consultation rate for depression, however, begins to fall in this age group (4th National Morbidity Study 1991–1992). Women in this age group may suffer adjustment reactions as a result of children leaving home, a change in employment and bereavement.

Old age. While the number of females consulting for depression decreases with age, the number of males complaining of depression increases. Severe depression is more common in the elderly than in younger age groups, the greatest risk of a first episode of severe depression occurring between 55 and 65 years of age.

Childhood. The incidence of emotional and psychological problems is on the increase among children and especially adolescents. Behaviour problems, school refusal and phobias may all have a basis in depression.

Presentation (Table 1)

Emotional symptoms. As the stigma of depression decreases in society, patients are increasingly likely to describe their symptoms and the probable cause of their depression. Some problems associated with depression may, however, go unmentioned. A loss of libido, which may occur early in the depression, may be a great source of interpersonal difficulty. Increased and excessive alcohol intake may similarly go unmentioned or may be revealed by the patient's partner as part of a briefing for the doctor.

Physical symptoms. Patients with ongoing or severe physical illness may suffer from depression. Those with depression will often describe physical symptoms such as weight loss, loss of appetite and energy, and chest and abdominal pains, which may all need investigation to rule out physical illness. Such patients may be unaware of any mood change or may attribute it simply to the physical symptoms. Physical symptoms may persist in the absence of physical signs and normal laboratory and radiology results. The presentation of physical symptoms as part of an underlying psychological illness being known as somatisation. Such patients may become increasingly anxious and

---

Table 1 **Common symptoms of depression**
■ Low self-esteem
■ Low mood
■ Nihilism – gloomy about the future
■ Worsening concentration
■ Suicidal ideation
■ Poor sleep
■ Appetite – too much or too little
■ Guilt
■ Irritability
■ Anxiety and panic attacks
■ Somatisation – aches and pains
■ Loss of libido

request referral to hospital. This often, however introduces them to a merry-go-round that puts them at risk of iatrogenic illness.

Males are more likely than females to present with somatic symptoms, as are people with a low IQ and those who are not psychologically literate.

Depression and suicide. Suicide is thankfully still uncommon, but its incidence is rising steadily in the Western world, now being about 13 per 100 000 population in England and Wales. In the younger age group, suicide is often an impulsive act while under the influence of alcohol. Antidepressants are implicated in 6.5% of suicides, the most dangerous period being the initial stages of treatment. Women usually select medication as their preferred method, while males tend to choose hanging.

Depression is an important risk factor in suicide (Table 2), but prescribing antidepressants for a patient who has suicidal ideation is a dilemma for GPs. Psychiatrists are frequently critical of GPs for under-treating depression, and it is known that a depressed patient who is suicidal is in need of urgent referral to a psychiatrist, but many patients express suicidal ideation that tends to settle with support, antidepressants and time. GPs tend to prescribe antidepressants for such patients on a weekly or two-weekly basis in order to keep an eye on them and to reduce the amount of harm should they overdose. Most governments now see suicide as an important public health and societal issue that needs to be urgently addressed.

Undetected depression. GPs diagnose and manage most depressed patients without referral to a psychiatrist, but GPs have been criticised for failing to recognise depression in a significant number of patients. A recent study involving 15 centres around the Western world (Wright 1999) studied the characteristics and outcomes of people with unrecognised depression. It was found that patients with unrecognised depression were younger and had had their symptoms for a shorter time than recognised patients. They also had less severe illness than recognised patients and lower suicidal and disability scores. Patients with unrecognised depression lost their symptoms at a rate similar to that of those with recognised depression. Although the study failed to show that the non-recognition of depression had a serious measurable effect, individuals in that group might still have benefitted from treatment (Wright 1999).

Doctors who are psychologically minded and who have good communication skills are more likely to detect depression. Interestingly, doctors who have themselves experienced depression are no more likely to detect it than those who have not suffered from it.

Management

Just because the GP may diagnose depression does not mean that the patient will agree with the diagnosis, particularly if the patient presents with somatic symptoms that cannot from their perspective be explained by a diagnosis of depression. Such a disagreement over diagnosis is unlikely to lead to compliance with treatment (British Journal of General Practice 1999). Even when the patient agrees with the doctor, there may, however, be a difference of opinion over the treatment of depression. GPs are known to favour medication, whereas patients may have reservations about antidepressants, fearing addiction, loss of control of their mind, or side-effects.

Because of the association of suicide with depression, it is important to assess the risk of suicide, but it is only in recent times that GPs have begun to ask patients about suicide as it was previously feared that such probing might put the idea into the patient's head. There are many ways of posing such an intimate and possibly intrusive question, and students and doctors need to become comfortable and unself-conscious when asking about suicide: 'Have your symptoms of unhappiness/misery ever made you think your life is not worth going on with' is a reasonably sensitive starting point. A surprising number of patients will have had fleeting ideas of escaping from their misery, but very few will have developed persistent ideas of suicide, and even fewer will admit to having made plans. Patients who made previous suicide attempts carry a higher risk (see Table 2).

When explaining the diagnosis of depression to a patient, it is important to emphasise that this is an illness. Patients, like doctors, may take a moral view of their depression, feeling that they need to 'pull themselves together'. Explaining that there may well be a deficiency of a chemical in the brain is a useful way of introducing the idea of antidepressant medication.

Two broad groups of antidepressants are currently in use: the older tricyclic antidepressants and the newer SSRIs. Both groups cause side-effects in approximately one third of patients, tricyclic antidepressants causing drowsiness, dryness of the mouth and blurred vision, and SSRIs causing gastrointestinal disturbances. Patients are often fearful that antidepressants are addictive, and it is well known that compliance is a general problem. There is uncertainty about how long patients need to take these medications, but a duration of 3–6 months is generally believed to achieve a good outcome.

Depression is sometimes rooted in childhood or social isolation, the support of the family, community psychiatric nurse and GP then being as important as medication in restoring the patient to good health. Counselling has a useful role to play in some patients, particularly if there are underlying psychological problems.

Recovery from depression, even with adequate medication is slow. In the Fifteen Cities study (Wright 1999), over half the patients taking antidepressants were still 'cases' of depression 1 year later. Similarly, 28% of those with unrecognised depression were still suffering from it 1 year later, as judged by questionnaires such as the General Health Questionnaire. Many people with a past history of depression will relapse at some stage in their lives.

While much depression is managed in general practice, referral to a psychiatrist is indicated if the diagnosis is uncertain, if there is a poor response to treatment or if there are psychotic features or a risk of suicide. Patients with psychomotor retardation and manic depression need referral to a psychiatrist.

Table 2 **Risk factors for suicide**
■ Previous parasuicide attempt
■ Increasing age
■ Male sex
■ Divorced/separated/living alone
■ Psychiatric illness
■ Economic distress
■ Alcohol/drug abuse

Common mental health problems II

Mood disorders *continued*

Bipolar disorder

In bipolar disorder, there will always be at least one attack of mania (Table 3) irrespective of whether or not depression has yet occurred. There is a prevalence rate of 4 per 1000, the incidence of bipolar disorder being higher in urban areas. The age of onset is in the late teens and early twenties, and there is an equal sex distribution. The lifetime risk for bipolar disorder in first-degree relatives is about 10%.

Course and prognosis

Before the advent of drugs such as chlorpromazine and lithium, the manic phase of bipolar disorder could last for months or even years. Death from exhaustion may occur in untreated mania. The risk of recurrence is over 50% if the disorder begins before the age of 30 years.

Treatment

The patient with mania usually needs admission to hospital, this sometimes needing to be compulsorily arranged. Those with lesser forms (hypomania) may be managed at home.

The care of a manic patient is a specialised nursing, medical, psychiatric and pharmacological process. About 50% of patients with bipolar disorder respond well to lithium, and there is good evidence for the effectiveness of lithium in the prevention of recurrent mood disturbances in patients with this disorder. The effectiveness of lithium is, however, reduced by poor compliance, alcohol and drug misuse, other psychiatric conditions and its side-effects.

Lithium is excreted largely unchanged in the kidney, which leads to lithium and sodium loss and both pose a risk of renal toxicity. Patients consequently need baseline renal function tests before starting lithium, followed by regular monitoring of the urea and electrolytes, creatinine and lithium levels while on medication.

Anxiety

Anxiety is a normal human response to new or stressful situations and a

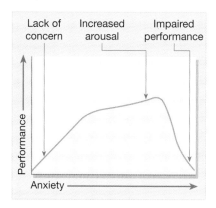

Fig. 1 **Yerkes–Dodson curve.**

part of the primitive 'fight or flight' reaction to danger. There is a relationship between performance and anxiety that is beneficial, but performance deteriorates when anxiety becomes pathological, as shown by the Yerkes–Dodson curve (Fig. 1).

Susceptibility to anxiety

Anxiety is a normal part of life but it becomes pathological when it interferes with a patient's life and decreases performance (Fig. 2).

- **Gender.** Over twice as many women as men consult their GP with anxiety. Unlike the situation with depression, the difference is consistent throughout all the age groups (4th National Morbidity Study 1991–1992). As in depression,

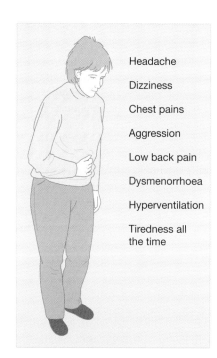

Headache

Dizziness

Chest pains

Aggression

Low back pain

Dysmenorrhoea

Hyperventilation

Tiredness all the time

Fig. 2 **Frequent complaints in anxiety.**

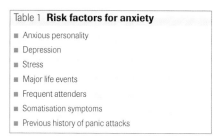

Table 1 **Risk factors for anxiety**

- Anxious personality
- Depression
- Stress
- Major life events
- Frequent attenders
- Somatisation symptoms
- Previous history of panic attacks

the figure quoted may not represent a true incidence of anxiety as men may resist seeing the doctor for their problems.

- **Personality.** Many people describe themselves as worriers and are habitually prone to anxiety (Table 1). A large proportion learn to accept it and live within its constraints by developing a way of life and relaxation that deals with their anxious nature.
- **Stress.** In some people, the anticipation of forthcoming stressful events can generate as much anxiety as the events themselves. Others put enormous efforts into coping with and containing their anxiety during stressful events, only to suffer afterwards. Events such as examinations, bereavement, moving house and relationship difficulties are common sources of anxiety.
- **Depression.** Most people with depression suffer some degree of anxiety, this being provoked by the feeling of social inadequacy and the fear of rejection that commonly accompany depression. Anxiety in depression may sometimes persist after the depression has lifted because of the lag in social recovery.
- **Physical illness.** Most illness and fear of illness is accompanied by anxiety. A physical illness in a patient who is pre-morbidly anxious is likely to worsen the anxiety. Snippets overheard on ward rounds or casual remarks made by doctors are mulled over by such patients and often make things worse.

Classes of anxiety

Psychiatrists have divided anxiety into three groups:

1. generalised anxiety disorder (formerly known as free-floating anxiety)
2. panic disorder
3. phobias.

Table 2 **Non-pharmacological methods for managing anxiety**
■ Reassurance
■ Exercise
■ Meditation
■ Reduction in caffeine and alcohol intake
■ Counselling

Table 3 **Features of mania**
■ Abnormally elevated mood
■ Irritability
■ Grandiosity
■ Boundless energy
■ Reduced sleep
■ Pressure of speech – over-talkative
■ Racing thoughts
■ Poor concentration – easily distracted
■ Hyperactivity, causing excessive spending of money/drinking/sexual activity

Source: Gelder et al (1996).

Generalised anxiety disorder

The patient complains of feeling tired all the time, jumpy and nervous, with light-headedness and dizziness. Patients often have a feeling of doom that either they or a family member will have a serious accident or contract a serious illness. More severe cases may have feelings of depersonalisation in which they feel that they are outside their body watching themselves. Physical symptoms include palpitations, sweating, headaches and indigestion.

Such patients are a challenge for general practice as their symptoms may suggest a variety of other illnesses. The GP will have to carry out laboratory tests in order to reassure both him- or herself and the patient. Most patients are grateful for negative results, and a discussion can then be opened up about their anxiety. Others with less insight may be confused by the negative results and demand further tests or referral.

As generalised anxiety disorder is likely to be lifelong, with exacerbations during stressful life events, treatment with benzodiazapines (such as diazepam) is hazardous; if these are to be used, closely monitored short courses are advised. Non-pharmacological methods of coping with anxiety (Table 2) are likely to be more helpful to the patient in the long term.

Panic disorder

Panic attacks are extremely frightening for patients in that they appear suddenly in an already anxious personality. A patient may get an attack of palpitations, sweating and hyperventilation. The attack may lead to collapse, the patient being rushed to the accident and emergency department. Panic attacks are unpredictable and their aetiology uncertain. Treatment is with tricyclic antidepressants rather than benzodiazapines.

Phobia

It is estimated that 5% of patients in general practice will have disabling phobias. However, only a minority of these will seek help. Indeed, patients may mention a phobia in passing as they have long learned to cope with it, usually by avoidance. Psychiatrists explain phobias in terms of classic conditioning: for example, a patient who has a dread of doctors will explain that she had a severe childhood illness that necessitated hospitalisation and many unpleasant procedures. Such patients may have a fear of all doctors or only of hospitals.

Agoraphobia is the most common phobia, the patient here having a fear of open spaces or of being enclosed. Patients can become completely housebound, being in the most severe cases unable to visit the doctor and requiring home visits for the most minor of illnesses. Agoraphobia occurs most frequently in women and begins in late adolescence or early adulthood.

Illness phobia or a fear of illness is common, but in a small number of people the fear dominates the patient's life, the medical profession being unable to provide reassurance. Such a phobia has much in common with an obsessional state and can sometimes be the presenting feature of depression.

Management

Most anxiety presenting in general practice needs nothing more than simple reassurance. If the patient has a particular anxiety about an illness, a laboratory or radiological test can be very comforting. Over-investigation may, however, reinforce the anxiety rather than relieve it.

Because anxiety and depression are intermingled, it is important to recognise and treat any underlying depression. GPs often give common-sense practical advice about life-style, which will include avoiding unnecessary stress, taking exercise and reducing coffee and alcohol intake.

Detailed interventions such as counselling are becoming more common in general practice. In addition, referral to a psychologist may be deemed necessary, especially for more disabling phobias.

Medication

A large number of benzodiazepines are prescribed and consumed annually. It is widely appreciated that these drugs are addictive and unsuitable over the long term, their use now beginning slowly to decline. It is thought that the maximum duration of treatment with benzodiazapines should be about 14 days.

Beta-blockers such as propranolol have been successful in treating anxiety. They are most useful in patients exhibiting somatic symptoms such as palpitations, and they are relatively safe. Psychiatrists prefer tricyclic antidepressants rather than anxiolytics to treat panic disorders.

Common mental health problems III

Schizophrenia

Schizophrenic-like illnesses have been recorded from ancient times, but the term 'schizophrenia' was first used in 1911 by Bleuler. Schizophrenia is a chronic relapsing and disabling illness that is now being treated less in long-term institutional care and more in the community. Community care is sometimes controversial and may be fragmented and indeed inappropriate.

Diagnosis

A diagnostic project in the USA and the UK (1972) pointed out a significant difference in the diagnosis of schizophrenia between the two countries. In the USA cases that would be diagnosed as depression, mania or personality disorder in the UK were called schizophrenia. The tighter the range of symptoms that are accepted as diagnostic of schizophrenia, the more reliable is the diagnosis, which led Kurt Schneider, founding father of psychiatry, to produce his list of so-called first rank symptoms of importance (Table 1). Even he, however, conceded that they do not always have to be present for a diagnosis to be made.

Estimates of the prevalence of schizophrenia depend on the criteria used for diagnosis. The annual incidence is probably between 0.1 and 0.5 per 1000 people and the lifetime risk of developing schizophrenia 7–9 per 1000 people. A GP with an average list size will thus have between 5 and 10 people with schizophrenia to look after.

The risk of a child developing schizophrenia is about 15% if one parent is schizophrenic and about 40% if both parents carry the diagnosis, providing clear evidence of a familial aetiology that may be attributable to the family environment rather than genetic factors.

Clinical features

In few other conditions do the features of the acute illness differ so much from those seen in the chronic illness (Table 2). Factors influencing outcome are listed in Table 3.

Management

The best results are obtained by combining drug and social treatments. The phenothiazine drugs (chlorpromazine, fluphenazine, and thioridazine) have an immediate calming and sedating effect on the patient but a slower anti-psychotic effect in the acute illness. The first effective drug to be used in the treatment of schizophrenia was chlorpromazine, but a wide range of similar medications is currently available, each with a different side-effect profile.

A significant minority of people with schizophrenia have, however, a resistance to phenothiazine-based medications. Clozapine achieves a good response in those who do not respond to traditional treatment, but

2% develop agranulocytosis in the first 18 weeks after starting treatment. Hence intensive white cell count checks are required early on and regularly thereafter. The powerful serotonin antagonist risperidone, without the haematological side-effects of clozapine, is also useful in treatment-resistant schizophrenia. Electroconvulsive therapy is reserved only for highly refractory cases.

Care in the community

The number of psychiatric beds in major institutions has decreased dramatically over the past 40 years because of a policy of moving people with chronic psychiatric problems into the community. This requires effective teamwork between agencies such as the medical social services, community psychiatric nurses and the patient and family. A keyworker is appointed who implements an agreed care plan. For community care to be successful, it needs inter agency co-operation with back-up from day-care centres, hostels and sheltered housing.

Case history

MJ is a 55-year-old woman with a history of schizophrenia. She was first admitted to a psychiatric hospital when aged 23, She lives with her elderly husband who has severe chronic obstructive pulmonary disease (COPD). She attends your practice weekly for repeat prescriptions of diazepam and anticholinergic medication. She is on long-term depot antipsychotic medication. This was previously administered by the community psychiatric nurse but last year MJ defaulted from care in the psychiatric services and now receives her depot medication from your practice. You can liase with the community psychiatric nurse if required.

Table 2 **Clinical features of acute and chronic schizophrenia**

Acute	Chronic
Delusions	Apathy
Hallucinations	Lack of drive
Interference with thinking	Slowness
	Social withdrawal

Table 1 **Schneider's symptoms of first-rank importance in the diagnosis of schizophrenia**

- Hearing thoughts spoken aloud
- Third-person hallucinations
- Hallucinations in the form of a commentary
- Somatic hallucinations
- Thought withdrawal or insertion
- Thought broadcasting
- Delusional perception
- Feeling that reactions are made or influenced by external agents

Table 3 **Factors predicting the outcomes of schizophrenia**

Good prognosis	Poor prognosis
Sudden onset	Insidious onset
No previous psychiatric history	Previous psychiatric history
Paranoid symptoms	Male gender
Older age at onset	Younger age onset
Good previous personality	Living alone
Good employment record	Poor pre-morbid personality
Good social networks	Unemployment
Good compliance with medication	Poor compliance with medication

Effects of schizophrenia on carers

The move to the community has caused particular difficulties for families. Patients with chronic schizophrenia suffer from social withdrawal, which means that they may not interact with other family members and may neglect themselves. Socially embarrassing behaviour brings patients to the attention of neighbours and the police, who will contact the family and the GP with the request that 'something must be done'. Relatives often feel anxious, depressed, guilty or helpless. They are often uncertain how to deal with difficult and odd behaviour, the stigma of mental illness discouraging open communication about the problem with friends and neighbours. This is a serious problem because good social and family networks are an important factor in good outcome for patients with schizophrenia.

Cognitive behavioural therapy

Cognitive behavioural therapy (CBT) is a psychological treatment that involves working with people to help them identify and deal with their problems.

It has been referred to as the 'talking cure'. It is used most commonly to treat patients with depression or anxiety though it is also used for many other conditions, such as eating disorders, chronic pain, chronic fatigue, personality disorders and schizophrenia. CBT is a collaborative treatment that can be offered at different levels of input from specialist treatment through to more focused interventions, such as self-help. It is frequently used in conjunction with medication and most commonly involves a course of between 6 and 20 1-hour treatment sessions.

Drug treatment

Chlorpromazine and haloperidol are long standing medications used for the control of psychotic symptoms. Their efficacy reaches a plateau whereas their frequent side-effects of sedation and extra pyramidal symptoms are dose related. The last decade has seen the emergence of new atypical antipsychotics that seek to be more effective against depressive and cognitive symptoms and that produce fewer extra pyramidal symptoms. A recent meta-analysis produced for the national schizophrenia guideline development group has concluded that there is no clear evidence that the newer antipsychotics are more effective or better tolerated than the older conventional antipsychotics. However, the meta-analysis did note that there are fewer extra pyramidal symptoms with the newer antipsychotics but recommended that conventional antipsychotics (chlorpromazine and haloperidol) should remain as the first line of treatment in schizophrenia.

Table 4
Conventional antipsychotic drugs
Chlorpromazine
Haloperidol
Newer antipsychotic drugs
Amisalpride
Chlozapine
Olanzapine
Quetiapine
Risperidone
Sertindole

References

www.mind.org.uk
www.babcp.com
www.nelh.nhs.uk.guidelines/
schizophrenia

Common mental health problems

- Ten per cent of those who consult their GP are depressed.
- Depression has biological, psychological, social and cultural features.
- Before modern pharmacology, mania could last for months and years.
- Anxiety and depression often occur together.
- While benzodiazepines are effective in anxiety, patients rapidly become dependent on them.
- Schizophrenia is a chronic relapsing disabling illness.
- The best outcomes in schizophrenia are obtained by a combination of pharmacological and social care.

Heart disease

The most common form of heart disease is ischaemic heart disease, or coronary artery disease (CAD). Other types include congenital heart disease, valvular defects and disorders of the myocardium or pericardium.

CAD is the largest cause of premature mortality in the developed world. In the UK, it is responsible for one third of male and a quarter of female deaths. Approximately 200 000 patients sustain a myocardial infarction in the UK every year. Half die from the infarction, and, of these, 50% do so before reaching hospital (Fig. 1). Although the incidence of CAD is falling slowly in developed countries (Fig. 1), it is increasing in Eastern Europe and other developing areas.

A GP with 2000 patients is likely to have 40 patients with CAD. In the course of 1 year, up to 12 of these will suffer a myocardial infarction.

Presentation

CAD can present in a number of ways (Table 1), the diagnosis being based largely on history.

Angina pectoris is the name given to the discomfort caused by transient myocardial ischaemia, the most common cause of which is CAD. Angina is characteristically described as a dull, tight, heaviness, pressure or discomfort in the centre of the chest, often precipitated by physical exertion, cold, intense emotion or a heavy meal. The pain can radiate into the neck, jaw, back and epigastrium or down the arms (usually the left) (Fig. 2) and is relieved by rest. Physical examination is usually normal.

Table 1 **Clinical Presentations of CAD**	
Clinical problem	**Pathology**
Stable angina	Ischaemia due to fixed atheromatous stenosis of one or more coronary arteries
Unstable angina	Ischaemia caused by dynamic obstruction of a coronary artery due to plaque rupture with superimposed thrombosis and spasm
Myocardial infarction	Acute occlusion of a coronary artery due to plaque rupture and thrombosis resulting in myocardial necrosis
Heart failure	Myocardial dysfunction due to infarction or ischaemia
Arrhythmias	Altered conduction due to ischaemia or infarction
Sudden death	Ventricular arrhythmia, asystole or massive acute myocardial infarction

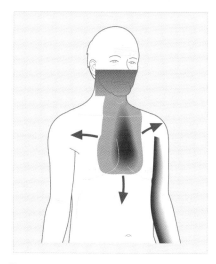

Fig. 2 **Diagram of distribution of pain in angina pectoris.**

In myocardial infarction, the pain is usually more severe and prolonged, lasting more than 15–20 minutes. It is often accompanied by shortness of breath, sweating, nausea or vomiting, light-headedness or tiredness. In severe cases, there can be syncope or collapse. Myocardial infarction is occasionally painless or 'silent', especially in elderly or diabetic patients.

Physical examination may reveal pallor, cyanosis, arrhythmia, hypertension and signs of cardiac failure.

Diagnosis

The diagnosis of angina or myocardial infarction is usually made on clinical findings, but further investigations are often indicated. Underlying or precipitating factors such as anaemia, hypothyroidism, diabetes mellitus and hyperlipidaemia should be excluded by the appropriate blood tests.

A resting ECG is normal in most cases of angina, but characteristic changes appear with myocardial infarction (Fig. 3). An exercise ECG involving a treadmill or bicycle is often required to confirm a diagnosis of angina and also gives some indication of the severity of CAD.

Myocardial infarction causes an elevation of cardiac enzymes, and serial measurement of these can be useful (Fig. 4).

A chest X-ray is often normal in myocardial infarction but can show evidence of cardiac failure. Other tests such as echocardiography and

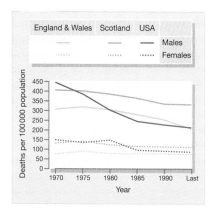

Fig. 1 **Deaths due to coronary artery disease in Scotland, England and Wales, and the USA in the years 1968–1992.**
(After Walker and Tan 2002.)

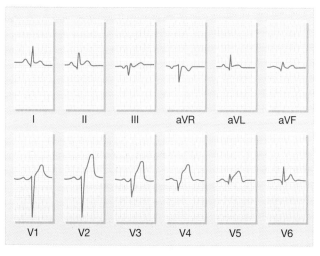

Fig. 3 **Characteristic ECG features of an acute anterior myocardial infarction.**
(After Walker and Tan 2002.)

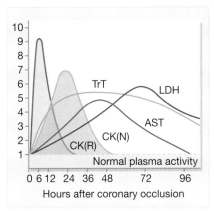

Fig. 4 **Changes in plasma enzyme concentrations after myocardial infarction.** CK: creatine kinase; TrT: troponin; AST: aspartate aminotransferase; LDH: lactate (hydroxybutyrate) dehydrogenase. CK and TrT are the first to rise, followed by AST and then LDH. In patients treated with a thrombolytic agent reperfusion is usually accompanied by a rapid rise in CK (curve CK(R), due to a washout effect; if there is no reperfusion, the rise is less rapid but the area under the curve is often greater (curve CK(N)). Source: Haslett et al (2003).

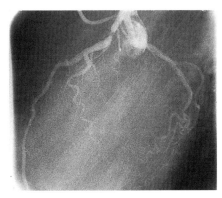

Fig. 5 **A coronary angiogram.** Note the severe stenosis of the left anterior descending coronary artery. Source: Haslett et al (2003).

radionuclide scanning tend to be used to detect complications such as valvular damage and pericardial effusions, and to assess left ventricular function.

Coronary angiography (Fig. 5) is used to define the nature and extent of CAD, usually prior to coronary artery bypass surgery or angioplasty.

Management

The management of angina involves advice on life-style and risk factor control (see below), medical measures and surgical treatment. Medical measures include the use of anti-anginal drugs and advice on avoiding precipitating factors. The three groups of drug used are:

- *nitrates*:
  – short acting, such as glyceryl trinitrate (sublingual or buccal)
  – long acting, such as isosorbide mononitrate
- *beta-adrenoceptor antagonists*, for example atenolol and metoprolol
- *calcium antagonists*, such as nifedipine and diltiazem.

Low-dose (75–300 mg) aspirin reduces the risk of myocardial infarction and cerebrovascular accident and should be taken by all patients with CAD unless contraindicated (allergy, known peptic ulcer or a bleeding disorder).

Surgical treatment includes percutaneous transluminal coronary angioplasty (PTCA) and coronary artery bypass grafting. The latter can not only relieve symptoms, but also prolong life expectancy. Coated metallic 'scaffolds' called stents can be inserted at the time of PTCA to maximise and maintain dilatation of the stenosed artery.

Myocardial infarction is usually best managed in a hospital coronary care unit because monitoring and resuscitation facilities are immediately available. Intravenous thrombolytics, for example streptokinase, can limit the extent of the infarction and significantly reduce mortality if given within the first few hours. Other early measures include bed rest, intravenous analgesia such as diamorphine, high-flow oxygen, anti-emetics (if required) and beta-adrenoceptor antagonists. In the absence of complications, patients can be mobilised by the second day

and discharged home within the week. Such patients can usually return to work within 6–8 weeks. Encouragement and active rehabilitation programmes seem to facilitate this process.

Risk factor control

A number of risk factors, some fixed and some modifiable, are associated with CAD (Table 2). Where appropriate, patients with CAD should be encouraged to stop smoking, take regular exercise, reduce saturated fat intake, maintain an ideal body weight and achieve a good control of any hypertension and diabetes (secondary prevention). Consideration should also be given to drug therapy with aspirin, β-blockers, ACE-inhibitors and lipid lowering agents. Primary prevention targetted at the whole population aims to combat CAD by modifying life-style factors such as smoking, diet and exercise before symptoms develop.

Prognosis

More than half of all patients with angina will live for 5 years and a third for 10 years from the time of diagnosis. Approximately 25% of patients with a myocardial infarction die within a few minutes. Half the deaths occur within 2 hours of the onset of symptoms and three-quarters within 24 hours. Of the survivors, 80% are still alive after 1 year, 75% after 5 and 50% after 10 years.

Table 2 **Risk factors for CAD**	
Fixed	**Modifiable**
Age	Smoking
Male sex	Hypertension
Family history	Lipid disorders
	Diabetes mellitus
	Haemostatic variables
	Sedentary life-style
	Obesity
	Dietary deficiences of antioxidant vitamins and polyunsaturated fatty acids

Heart disease

- Coronary artery disease (CAD) is the most common form of heart disease, accounting for one third of male and one quarter of female deaths in UK.
- A GP with 2000 patients is likely to have 40 patients with CAD.

- CAD involves multiple risk factors, some fixed and some modifiable.
- Modifiable factors include smoking, hypertension, hyperlipidaemia, diabetes mellitus, a lack of exercise, obesity and polyunsaturated fatty acid deficiencies.

- The clinical presentation of CAD ranges from mild chest pain through to sudden death. Good history-taking is the key to diagnosis.
- The management of angina involves advice on life-style and risk factor control, medical

measures and sometimes surgical treatment.

- Myocardial infarction is usually best managed in a hospital coronary care unit.
- More than half of all patients will live for 5 years and a third for 10 years from the time of diagnosis.

Chronic musculoskeletal disorders

Up to 15% of people consult their GP annually for musculoskeletal problems. The figure increase dramatically with age, although attributing musculoskeletal illness to 'old age' frustrates patients and may lead them unnecessarily to restrict their activities. Four common musculoskeletal conditions form the bulk of work in general practice are:

- osteoarthritis
- rheumatoid arthritis
- low back pain
- fibromyalgia.

Osteoarthritis

This is a major cause of pain, disability and loss of function that affects more than 15% of the population aged over 55 years in the UK. It is the result of a 'wear and tear' process that is characterised by a loss of cartilage with a hypertrophic bony response (Table 1). It affects significantly more females than males, osteoarthritis of the hip especially being more common among Caucasians.

Obesity is a risk factor for both genders but more so for females. Arthritis and obesity go hand in hand as arthritis limits exercise, which in turn deprives patients of a vital mechanism for controlling their weight. Increasing weight in turn leads to greater pressure on the weight-bearing joints, contributing to additional wear and tear.

There is a positive family history in osteoarthritis, physically demanding occupations such as farming also increasing the incidence. Contact sports are also associated with the condition, soccer players, for example, showing injuries to their ankles and knees. Similarly, sports men or women and others who undergo

meniscectomy for a knee injury are left with an increased risk of osteoarthritis in the affected joint.

Clinical features

Patients attribute most aches and pains in their joints to arthritis, most also blaming the weather – the wet weather in temperate climates and the hot weather in sunnier climes. In general practice, most patients with joint or neck pain will eventually request an X-ray, which will not usually, much to the patient's surprise, reveal any abnormality. By the time that radiological evidence is present, the arthritis is well advanced. Orthopaedic surgeons are better able to establish the nature and state of the pathology by arthroscopic visualisation of the joint.

The clinical symptoms of osteoarthritis (Table 2) are mainly pain and crepitus in the affected joint, with stiffness and associated loss of function. The pain may be continuous and worse after weight-bearing use, which limits the patient's ability to get about, leading to weight gain. Pain may be referred: osteoarthritis of the hip may, for example, present as knee pain. Decreased use through pain leads to muscle wasting around the affected joint, which may lead to the joint suddenly giving way. This is often evident in the knee joint, where lack of use is known to lead to wasting of the quadriceps in days in acute cases.

More advanced arthritis leads to joint thickening, which is clinically evident in, for example, the knee. The patient experiences lack of movement and flexibility, which is further limited by pain.

The hip and knee joints are commonly affected in osteoarthritis. Arthritis in the knees is usually bilateral, the patient being more likely to be obese and female; in the hip

joint, the condition is common in those with a history of Perthes' disease or trauma.

Diagnosis

The diagnosis of osteoarthritis is based on the history and physical examination, radiology not generally being recommended as part of the routine diagnosis. An X-ray will typically reveal a loss of joint space with osteophyte formation.

Management

It is important to keep the patient mobile by relieving the pain and reducing inflammation. There is concern that some anti-inflamatory medications actually exacerbate the destruction of especially the hip joints. The advice of a physiotherapist who can teach appropriate exercises and encourage the patient to be mobile is important.

Weight reduction is a problem that many people disabled by osteorthritis find difficult, some insoluble, but a dietary review can be helpful here. Patients often seek their doctor's advice on exclusion diets that may give them unreasonable expectations of improvement or cure.

Sensible footwear, especially on uneven ground, is beneficial; patients seem to resort to a stick only when they have moderate difficulty with support and mobility. Surgery also has a valuable and highly valued role in osteoarthritis, especially of the hip and to a lesser extent of the knee. Patients describe the relief of pain as liberating them to return to a mobile, almost normal life.

Rheumatoid arthritis

The point prevalence of rheumatoid arthritis is about 1%, the condition being three times more common in women than men. It is a disease worth studying as patients with rheumatoid arthritis often appear in clinical examinations. Patients with chronic rheumatoid arthritis are seen about three times a year in general practice for many years as their life expectancy is often normal and their care is increasingly shared with the rheumatologist. Although rheumatoid arthritis is a chronic systemic inflammatory disorder affecting predominantly the musculoskeletal

Table 1 **Determinants of osteoarthritis**
■ Increasing age
■ Gender – 50% increase in females
■ Caucasian race – especially osteoarthritis of the hip
■ Obesity – odds ratio 4.5 for men, 9 for women
■ Positive family history of nodal arthritis
■ Mechanical factors
■ Some occupations, e.g. farming
■ Post-injury
■ Some contact sports
■ Post-meniscectomy

Table 2 **Signs of osteoarthritis**
■ Crepitus in the joints
■ Increase in bony thickness
■ Deformity
■ Instability of joint: 'gives way'
■ Decreased movement
■ Pain especially on moving
■ Muscle wasting, especially in the quadriceps

Table 3 **Criteria for the diagnosis of rheumatoid arthritis (American Rheumatism Association/American College of Rheumatology 1987): at least four criteria must be fullfilled**

Criteria	Comment
Morning stiffness	Duration greater than 1 hour lasting longer than 6 weeks
Arthritis in at least three areas[1]	Soft tissue swelling lasting longer than 6 weeks
Arthritis of hand joints	Wrist, metacarpophalangeal joints or proximal interphalangeal joints lasting longer than 6 weeks
Symmetrical arthritis	At least one area lasting longer than 6 weeks
Rheumatoid nodules (occur in 30% of patients)	Especially in the elbows and buttocks
Positive rheumatoid factor	A negative test does not exclude disease
X-ray changes	Especially in the wrist and hands

[1]Proximal interphalangeal joints, metacarpophalangeal joints, wrist/elbow/knee/ankle and metatarsophalangeal joints

Table 4 **Laboratory diagnosis of rheumatoid arthritis**

- Raised erythrocyte sedimentation rate
- Increased C-reactive protein level
- Rheumatoid factor
- Positive X-rays

Table 5 **Joints commonly affected in rheumatoid arthritis**

Finger	40%
Shoulder	20%
Foot	20%
Wrist	15%
Knee	3%
Nodules of forearms, buttocks, lungs	30%

Source: Eberhardt (1990)

Table 6 **Common non-articular manifestations of rheumatoid arthritis**

Lymph node enlargement	50%
Splenomegaly	25%
Pleuritis	30%
Pericarditis	10%
Myositis	Common
Muscle atrophy	Common
Osteoporosis	Common
Sjögren's syndrome	10%
Nerve entrapment	Common

system, there are also important and disabling extra-articular manifestations.

Diagnosis

The diagnosis is based on a combination of clinical and laboratory observations that have been standardised by various learned colleges and associations (Tables 3 and 4).

Unlike osteoarthritis, rheumatoid arthritis favours the small joints of the hand and largely spares the weight-bearing hip and knee joints (Table 5). A large proportion of patients develop nodules on the ulnar aspects of their forearms, over their ischial tuberosities and in their lungs (Caplan's syndrome).

Some of the bewildering array of extra-articular manifestations have been quantified, others commonly being seen as part of clinical experience. Although some may be symptomless, others may cause serious and painful problems such as pericarditis, osteoporosis and nerve entrapment (Table 6).

Management

Many patients with rheumatoid arthritis experience functional deterioration after about 15 years. Rheumatologists, often in partnership with GPs, are adopting an increasingly aggressive and optimistic approach to rheumatoid arthritis. Reducing pain and limiting inflammation are both mainstays of reducing the disability of the condition.

Non-steroidal inflammatory agents (NSAIDs) are the first-line agents. Gold and penicillamine are commonly used second-line that modify disease, but their side-effects have to be carefully monitored. Methotrexate, azathioprine and cyclophosphamide are immunosuppressive drugs reserved for third-line therapy. Surgery has a role in joint replacement, plastic hand surgery being increasingly used. As the therapy is aggressive in rheumatoid arthritis, management of the side-effects, and of disease effects such as anaemia and vasculitis, is important.

Low back pain

See p. 79.

Fibromyalgia

This is a relatively common non-articular rheumatic condition causing chronic diffuse musculoskeletal pain, non-restorative sleep and fatigue. It is also associated with tenderness at specific reproducible locations known as tender spots or trigger points, of which there are a total of 18, corresponding to the acupuncture points for pain relief. Trigger points are characterised by local tenderness that becomes worse and may be referred elsewhere on examination.

Fibromyalgia is five times more common in women than in men and is aggravated by cold, humidity, tension, fatigue or too much or too little activity.

Diagnosis

Fibromyalgia may mimic other diseases of musculoskeletal or cardiac origin. The diagnosis is made mainly on the history and on positive trigger points, the usual laboratory tests being normal albeit reassuring for the patient. Aggravating psychological factors are important in around 25% of patients.

Management

The trigger points are surprisingly resistant to analgesia and NSAIDs, although low-dose antidepressants are beneficial in some cases. Patients benefit from knowing the chronic nature of the disorder and can institute a regime of exercise and stress management with some benefit. They may require ongoing support and reassurance.

Chronic musculoskeletal disorders

- Nearly 1 in 5 people consult their GP with aches and pains.
- Increasing age, obesity and occupation are important factors in osteoarthritis.
- Patients with rheumatoid arthritis often appear in clinical examinations.
- Fibromyalgia is common in general practice and 25% of patients have aggravating psychological problems.

Chronic back and neck pain

Man's erect posture places considerable mechanical stress on the vertebral spine and its associated structures. The weakest parts of the spine are at its points of maximum curvature, in the neck and lower back. Although there are other important causes of chronic back or neck pain mechanical causes are the most common. The structures involved are shown in Fig. 1.

Aetiology

Spondylosis

'Spondylosis' is the term loosely used to describe the degenerative changes that occur with increasing age in the cervical and lumbar regions, narrowing the spinal canal, especially around the C4–5, C5–6 and C6–7 regions in the neck and L4–5 and L5–S1 regions in the lower back. Pain may occur purely around the spine, without any referred (root) pain, arising from the degenerative changes themselves (akin to osteoarthritis being caused by the 'wear and tear' process).

Degenerative change 'hardens' the gel-like properties of the healthy nucleus pulposus, so that, instead of distributing pressure equally, points of high pressure develop. Intra-disc pressure is increased by lifting, especially while bending forwards or sitting. Disc protrusion usually occurs posterolaterally because that is where support structures are weakest. If a nerve root is compressed by the disc protrusion, there will be pain and paraesthesiae in the corresponding cutaneous distribution of the nerve segment (Fig. 2).

Prolapsed invertebral disc

In general, back pain is common in most adult age groups (although the causes may be different), but pain in the neck is mostly caused by spondylosis, occurring principally in the elderly. Although prolapsed intervertebral disc lesions occur more easily in older spondylytic spines, younger people may subject themselves to a greater risk of mechanical injury, so that prolapsed disc occurs quite commonly from late teenage years onwards (Table 1).

Myelopathy

The spinal cord ends at the L2 level, so disc protrusion at the lumbar level can generally affect only nerve roots (including the cauda equina, see

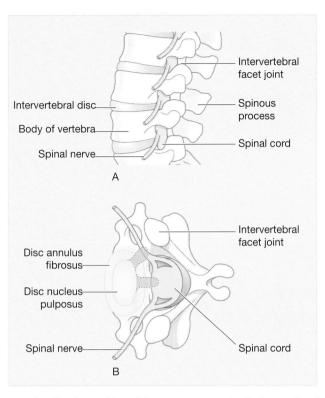

Fig. 1 **Diagram showing the position of the nerve roots and spinal nerve in relation to skeletal structures. (A)** Lateral aspect of the lumbar spine. **(B)** Superior aspect of a cervical vertebra. The precise position of the union of the ventral and dorsal nerve roots, to form the spinal nerve, in the intervertebral foramen is a little variable. Dotted lines indicate the usual sites of disc herniation.

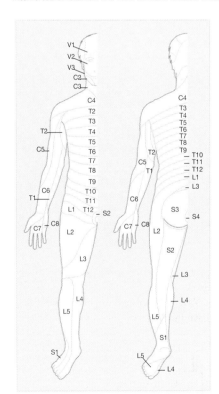

Fig. 2 **Dermatome chart (left: anterior; right: posterior).** A dermatome is an area of skin supplied by one segmental sensory nerve. The dermatomes overlap, and variations can be expected.

Table 1 **Causes of low back pain related to specific age groups**	
Age group (years)	**Cause of pain**
Children	Osteochondrosis (Scheuermann's disease)
	Scoliosis – primary or secondary
18–30	Ankylosing spondylitis
	Prolapsed invertebral disc and fractures
	Spondylolisthesis
	Postural pain from pregnancy
30–50	Degenerative joint disease
	Prolapsed invertebral disc
	Malignancy
50 and over	Degenerative joint disease
	Osteoporosis
	Paget's disease
	Malignancy

below), rather than the spinal column itself. At cervical level, however, it is possible (but fortunately rare) for disc protrusion to compress the spinal cord, giving rise to a classical syndrome of upper motor neurone signs of spastic paraparesis in the lower limbs (as a result of cord compression) with lower motor neurone signs in the upper limbs (due to nerve root compression).

Other causes

Table 1 also shows some of the main non-mechanical causes of back and neck pain (particularly back pain). Although most of these are much less common, they need to be identified at

Table 2 Clinical features of low back pain

Feature	History	Examination
Mechanical	Precipitating strain Previous episodes Unilateral leg/buttock pain Worse on movement and coughing Eased by rest	Assymmetrical restriction of movement and of straight leg raising Uniradicular signs
Systemic disease	Constant or progressive Worse on rest or at night Morning stiffness Bilateral or alternating pain Diffuse pain and tenderness	Features of ill-health Rigid lumbar spine Symmetrical restriction of movement and straight leg raising Multiradicular signs Other neurological signs Wasting of paraspinal muscles High ESR
Non-specific	Postural factors Depression Gynaecological symptoms Diffuse pain	Normal movement Local tenderness

an early stage because different management will be required. Table 2 shows the main clinical features.

Clinical features

Psychological and social factors

Simple postural factors, such as a bad posture, bad chair design, a lack of training in lifting procedures, a lack of exercise and prolonged travel in badly designed vehicles are thought to be the most common causes of backache. Chronic low back pain in particular may also be caused or prolonged by unhappiness at work or at home, often as a result of complex factors that may be difficult to identify. Much back pain is related to occupation or caused by accidents in the workplace, when the possibility of compensation or early retirement because of ill-health may be an additional factor.

Low back pain is one of the most common causes of dysfunction and loss of working time. It often requires an especially holistic approach, and it is most important to help the patient to avoid the prolonged and intractable disability that may arise when important psychosocial factors are not identified at an early stage.

Neck pain

Pain caused by cervical degenerative arthritis (spondylosis) is extremely common in the middle aged and elderly. Although there may be some transient associated nerve root irritation, with pain in the shoulder, upper arm and occasionally lower arm and hand on the affected side, there are no neurological signs. More persistent or severe root pain suggests cervical radiculopathy, caused by narrowing of the exit foramina for the nerve root from the spine, combined with disc degeneration and a loss of disc space height.

The pain is aggravated by coughing or sneezing, which transiently raises intraspinal (CSF) pressure. At this stage, there may be weakness of the shoulder and upper arm muscles (deltoid, spinati and biceps), with diminished biceps and supinator reflexes; myelopathy, although it is very unusual, must be positively excluded. Referral for investigation may be needed. Surgery is fortunately only very rarely required, the usual treatment being analgesia and a cervical collar.

Low back pain

Each year, about 5% of the population have low back pain, and over a lifetime, almost everyone has had it at some time. The identification of an anatomical diagnosis is difficult and (fortunately) unnecessary in most cases (Table 2). In 9 out of 10 cases, the precise cause is never identified, and the patient is back to work within 3 months, four out of five patients being back to work in less than a month. These patients will have had some form of mechanical injury to the back. Recent evidence suggests that prolonged rest is not beneficial but that patients should keep mobile, perhaps helped by analgesia and back exercises.

About 1% of patients with back pain have lumbosacral radiculopathy or sciatica, with pain radiating down one leg. Note that pain in the leg does not by itself indicate root pain – it may also occur with straight forward musculoskeletal injury. Most commonly, the L5 root is compressed by prolapse of the L4–5 disc, with pain in the lateral aspect of the leg and dorsum of the foot; alternatively, the S1 root may be compressed by an L5–S1 prolapse, with pain down the back of the leg to the sole of the foot. As with cervical radiculopathy, the pain is aggravated by coughing or sneezing.

Because the nerve root is trapped by the disc, stretching the root by the straight leg raising test causes pain and is a good measure of severity as well as of the progress of treatment. If the sciatica is also reproduced by raising the opposite leg, the diagnosis of prolapsed disc is even more likely. In three out of four patients, the sciatic pain is almost gone within 2–4 weeks, using the same management as for non-sciatic back pain.

The diagnostic distinction of prolapsed disc from other mechanical causes of low back pain is therefore relatively unimportant for management unless the pain persists and surgical treatment has to be contemplated.

Alarm bells

Apart from malignancy and major neurological involvement caused by pressure on the spinal cord (see text), the main danger situation is acute central disc prolapse in the lumbar area (fortunately uncommon). This occur when the disc protrudes in the midline, compressing the cauda equina. The main signs are:

- bilateral nerve signs (e.g. both legs)
- a disturbance of micturition
- a loss of sensation in the perineal area ('saddle anaesthesia')

Urgent surgery is needed to prevent permanent bowel and bladder incontinence.

Chronic back and neck pain

- Man's erect posture puts great mechanical strain on the weakest parts of the spine – the neck and lower back.

- Progressive 'wear and tear' damages the vertebral structures and may cause chronic pain in the neck or back.

- However, the most common causes are bad posture, lack of exercise, obesity and other mechanical factors.

- Psychological and social factors play a part, particularly in prolonging symptoms.

- Other causes of back pain, such as systemic disease, are relatively rare but often potentially serious – some of the 'danger signs' are listed.

Urinary tract problems

An estimated 11% of patients consult their GP at least once for a genitourinary complaint. Except for children under the age of 5, the consultation rate is much higher among females than males (Fig. 1). The sex difference is very pronounced between the ages of 16 and 64, females consulting 12 times more frequently than males. This predominance among women is caused by the female susceptibility to urinary tract infections (UTIs). Age increases the prevalence of urinary symptoms especially in men (Fig. 1).

Children

Urinary tract infections

Many UTIs in children are asymptomatic, an incidence of asymptomatic infection in girls aged 14–16 of up to 2% being reported. Girls are more frequently affected than boys, and urinary infection is clinically more damaging in children under the age of 4 years. Renal scarring may occur, which impairs renal growth, and scarring before the age of 4 years can progress if the infection is not controlled. Over one third of children with a UTI show some degree of vesico-ureteric reflux.

Diagnosis. Presentation is often with non-specific symptoms of fever, common malaise, vomiting or failure to thrive. Older children may present with enuresis or specific symptoms related to the urinary tract.

Management. Antibiotic treatment for up to 1 week will clear

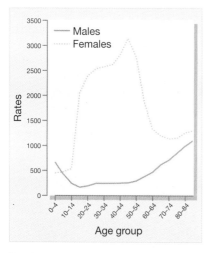

Fig. 1 **Patient consulting rates 1:10 000 person years at risk.** Source: 4th National Morbidity study 1991–2 OPCS.

most infections. However, particularly before the age of 4, investigation may be necessary to detect reflux, scarring or renal abnormality. Children with reflux or recurrent infection may need regular prophylactic antibiotics, which are extremely effective in preventing further scarring. The natural history of reflux is for resolution in the majority of children; only a minority will go on to need surgery, which includes re-implantation of the ureters.

Enuresis

Between 10% and 20% of 5-year-olds and 5–10% of 10-year-olds wet their bed at night, and the problem may persist into adulthood. Unlike UTIs, enuresis is more common in boys and in social classes IV and V.

UTIs are found in up to 10% of children with enuresis. For many children presenting with nocturnal enuresis there, is, however, no obvious social, psychological or organic disturbance. Such children probably represent the tail end of normal development. Enuresis is sometimes seen in association with life events such as a new baby in the family, or starting school. Nowadays, child sex abuse has also to be considered as a cause.

A good history explores whether the child has always been wet at night (primary enuresis) or whether there have been precipitating events (secondary enuresis). The reaction of the child and parents to the enuresis is important, as is the ritual that may develop concerning the disposal of bed linen, the night-wear worn and social restrictions. Physical examination is carried out largely to reassure the family, and a mid-stream urine (MSU) for laboratory examination is essential to rule out an infection.

Management. There is a strong placebo effect in the doctor's interest in the patient, and a simple star chart that rewards dry nights will sort out most children. Some need an alarm that is activated by the urine. A surprising number of children, however, sleep through the alarm, even though it manages to wake everyone else in the house. The antidepressants imipramine and amitryptiline in a low dose have been shown to be effective in the treatment of enuresis. The anti-diuretic hormone desmopressin, an analogue of

vasopressin, is also used for nocturnal enuresis for a period of 3 months.

Women

Urinary tract infections

The shortness of the female urethra is believed to be the cause of the problem here. During sexual intercourse, organisms track up the urethra and into the bladder to cause infection. Post-coital micturition reduces the risk of UTI.

Usual presentations. Whereas childhood urinary infections present as non-specific illness, the diagnosis being made only on urine culture, older children and adults – both women and men – present with frequency, dysuria, nocturia and, less commonly, loin pain and systemic upset.

Diagnosis. In young children, the diagnosis is only made if the physician thinks of obtaining an MSU from an unwell child with non-specific symptoms, but in adults, the history is the cornerstone of diagnosis, this being confirmed by an MSU. In the doctors' surgery, the urine can be tested by dipsticks that can detect the presence of blood, nitrites and leukocytes.

The microscopy of fresh unspun urine is also very helpful and may, under a high-powered field, reveal the presence of pus cells. Microscopy is more commonly carried out in mainland Europe than in the UK, but laboratory diagnosis is the gold standard. Finding more than 10^5 organisms per ml of urine is considered to be diagnostic of a UTI. Most UTIs are caused by enteric organisms, *Escherichia coli* being responsible for about 85% of cases; less commonly, *Klebsiella* and *Proteus* are detected.

Management. UTIs in non-pregnant women between the ages of 16 and 65 are usually uncomplicated as investigations rarely reveal an underlying cause. The management of an uncomplicated UTI is:

- increased fluid intake
- regular bladder emptying
- antibiotics.

Antibiotics may be given as large single-dose therapy or as therapy for 3–5 days. The antibiotic of choice is usually trimethoprim because it is active against the usual urinary organisms, has a long duration of action and is excreted unchanged in the urine. It can be given twice daily.

Men

Urinary tract infections

UTI is not as common in males as in females, except during the neonatal phase. A UTI in a male is often associated with genitourinary abnormalities, investigation being warranted. UTIs in older males are generally related to prostatic obstruction (see p. 49).

Urinary symptoms in prostatism

(see also p. 49)

All too often, the presentation is to the GP of an older male with a UTI, or to the accident and emergency department of an elderly man who has gone into urinary retention. The symptoms of a UTI are the same for men as for women. Older males presenting with urinary symptoms need to have further investigations in the urology department as the underlying problem is usually prostatic in origin.

Benign prostatic hypertrophy is described as either obstructive or irritative:

- *Obstructive.* This is caused by narrowing of the urethra by the enlarging prostate. The symptoms include:
  - hesitancy
  - a weak stream
  - straining
  - prolonged micturition
  - a feeling of incomplete emptying
  - overflow incontinence.
- *Irritative.* This is caused by irritable bladder muscle as a result of high voiding pressures and incomplete emptying. The symptoms include:
  - nocturia
  - daytime frequency
  - urgency
  - urge incontinence.

Despite the high prevalence of benign prostatic hypertrophy, most men do not seek help from their GP or urologist for the condition. There are many reasons for this, including embarrassment, a fear of surgical treatment, a fear of prostate cancer and an acceptance that it is merely a sign of old age.

General urinary conditions

Recurrent urinary tract infections

Many women suffer from recurrent uncomplicated UTIs, needing prompt antibiotic treatment together with an increased fluid intake at the onset of symptoms. They also benefit from emptying the bladder after intercourse.

Complicated urinary tract infections

Complicated UTIs occur in children, pregnant women, and men.

Men and children under 5 years of age presenting with a UTI require additional investigations because there may well be an underlying abnormality of the genitourinary tract. Asymptomatic bacteriuria occurs in about 5% of non-pregnant women and does not usually cause any difficulty. If, however, a patient with asymptomatic bacteriuria becomes pregnant, she runs an increased risk of developing a UTI with pyelonephritis. Women in early pregnancy should ideally, have an MSU, but failing that, lower urinary tract symptoms have to be dealt with promptly because of the risk of pyelonephritis and the threat of prematurity for the fetus.

Incontinence of urine

This is defined as an involuntary loss of urine during the day or night; a prevalence of over 50% has been reported among nursing students in America. In general practice, the overall prevalence among women is found to be 41%. However, only about one third of women worry about their incontinence, and of these less than one third discuss their problem with their GP or district nurse. There are two types of incontinence – stress urinary incontinence and detrusor instability – although these can co-exist.

Stress urinary incontinence. This occurs when the bladder pressure exceeds the maximum urethral closure pressure. It is common in multiparous women as vaginal delivery can result in a decrease of urethral closure function. It occurs on coughing, laughing, jogging and is accompanied by the repeated loss of a small amount of urine.

The majority of patients with stress urinary incontinence show an improvement with conservative treatment such as physiotherapy and medication. The basis of physiotherapy is teaching patients to use their pelvic floor muscles to enable better urinary control. Alpha- or beta-adrenergic drugs are also used; these cause the urethra and bladder neck to contract.

There are over a hundred different surgical procedures for stress urinary incontinence, involving buttressing the bladder, colposuspension, the formation of a bladder sling and elevation of the bladder neck with a nylon sling.

Detrusor instability. This is an impairment of voluntary control of the bladder and is present in about 10% of the adult population. It is important to distinguish detrusor instability from stress urinary incontinence as the basis of the management of detrusor instability is medical and behavioural, whereas in stress incontinence surgery has a role.

The symptoms of detrusor instability are both diurnal and nocturnal frequency, urgency and urge incontinence. However, stress and urge incontinence co-exist in about 20% of patients. There is a strong association between both neurotic personality traits and anxiety and both detrusor instability and stress urinary incontinence.

Whereas stress urinary incontinence can be replicated clinically by asking the patient to cough, diagnosing detrusor instability needs an MSU to exclude infection, and then cystometry and cystoscopy.

The drug management of detrusor instability involves anticholinergic drugs such as oxybutynin. Bladder drill is the favourite behavioural therapy; this involves retraining the bladder and trying to separate micturition from the anticipation of urgency and incontinence. Surgically, cystocopy and urethral dilatation are also used.

Urinary tract problems

- Females suffer more urinary symptoms but age increases the symptomatology in both sexes.
- UTIs in children are a hidden problem.
- The presentation of benign prostatic hypertrophy is sometimes an older man in acute retention.
- Incontinence of urine is very common but only a minority seek medical advice.

Epilepsy

Epilepsy encompasses a group of disorders in which there are recurrent episodes of altered cerebral function associated with a paroxysmal excessive electrical discharge of the neurones. The clinical manifestation of these episodes – fits, seizures or convulsions – range from transient, minor 'absences' to prolonged major convulsions with a loss of consciousness, incontinence and limb jerking. The different types of fit are shown in Table 1.

A GP with 2000 patients can expect 1–2 new cases annually, 10–15 patients with epilepsy consulting and another 40–50 persons with a past history but no current problems. Epilepsy can start at any age but is most likely in children. Males and females are equally affected.

In the majority of cases, no cause can be found (idiopathic epilepsy), but in up to 40% of these patients, there is a family history of epilepsy in a close relative; this is often the case with petit mal. The causes of epilepsy are shown in Table 2.

Table 1 **Type of fit**	
General seizures	Grand mal
	Absence (petit mal)
	Akinetic or atonic
	Myoclonic
Partial (focal) seizures	Simple (awareness preserved)
	– Motor
	– Sensory
	– Psychomotor
	– Visual
	– Versive
	Complex (awareness lost)
	– Temporal
	– Frontal

Table 2 **Causes of epilepsy**
■ Hereditary and familial factors
■ Developmental defects (intra-uterine rubella, phakomatoses)
■ Birth trauma
■ Anoxia in infancy and childhood
■ Head injury
■ Tumours (primary and secondary)
■ Infection (febrile convulsions, meningitis or encephalitis)
■ Vascular accidents or malformations
■ Inflammation (systemic lupus erythematosus, polyarteritis nodosa and multiple sclerosis)
■ Metabolic disorders (hypoglycaemia, uraemia or hypocalcaemia)
■ Toxins (alcohol and drugs)
■ Degenerative disorders (Alzheimer's disease and Creutzfeldt–Jakob disease)

Table 3 **Factors provoking fits**
■ Infections and pyrexia
■ Physical and mental exhaustion
■ Sleep deprivation
■ Emotional stress
■ Drug or alcohol ingestion or withdrawal
■ Flickering lights, visual patterns and proximity to TV screens

In some cases, certain factors can provoke fits (see Table 3)

Presentation
The different types of fit present in different ways, but there may be a mixture in individuals (Fig. 1).

Generalised fits
These include the following:

■ **Grand mal.** This type is sometimes preceded by a prodromal phase of unease and irritability. There may be an aura (olfactory hallucination, or déjà vu) before the tonic phase, in which there is sustained muscular contraction that may be associated with a 'cry', cyanosis, tongue-biting and incontinence (lasting 10–30 seconds). The clonic phase (lasting 1–5 minutes) follows, with repeated violent, jerking movements that may result in self-injury.

Finally, in the post-ictal phase, the patient passes from deep unconsciousness with flaccid limbs through a stuporous phase that can be associated with headache, drowsiness, confusion and sometimes automatic behaviour and amnesia (lasting a few minutes to several hours).

■ **Petit mal.** These are brief (10–15 second) absence attacks with some alteration in consciousness during which the child ceases activity,

stares, rolls up the eyes or flutters the eyelids

■ **Akinetic or atonic fits.** These are sudden, transient losses of muscle tone leading to a fall.

■ **Myoclonic fits.** These are sudden brief episodes of generalised muscle twitching but no altered consciousness.

Partial fits
These include the following types:

■ *Motor.* A convulsive twitching of one side of the body, often starting in the face or hand and gradually spreading (Jacksonian epilepsy). This is sometimes followed by a transient monoparesis (Todd's paralysis).

■ *Sensory.* A spread similar to Jacksonian epilepsy but only tingling or 'electric' sensations.

■ *Psychomotor.* Déjà vu, unusual smells, emotional changes, lip-smacking, hallucinations of sounds, smell, taste or vision, and aimless or automatic behaviour.

■ *Visual.* Hallucinations in the form of balls of light, coloured patterns, faces or scenes.

■ *Versive.* The eyes and head are turned to one side.

■ *Temporal.* The most common type of partial seizure. Olfactory, epigastric and psychic phenomena are very common and may be accompanied by repetitive motor behaviour.

■ *Frontal.* Similar to temporal fits but arising from the frontal lobes.

Febrile fits
These are usually brief, generalised and associated with fever in children between 6 months and 5 years or age, peaking at between 9 months and

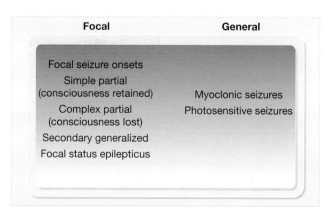

Fig. 1 **Seizure types in focal and generalized epilepsies.** Adapted from Fuller

Table 4 **Key diagnostic features of epilepsy**
■ A family history of epilepsy
■ Factors that may provoke fits (see Table 3)
■ A prodromal phase or aura/hallucinations
■ Tonic/clonic movements
■ Tongue-biting and incontinence
■ Salivation and cyanosis
■ Altered or loss of consciousness, and falling down
■ Post-ictal symptoms such as headache and drowsiness
■ Automation

Table 5 **Immediate care for a seizure: first aid**
■ Move the person away from any danger (fire, water, machinery or furniture)
■ After the convulsions cease, turn the patient into the 'recovery' position (semi-prone)
■ Ensure the airway is clear
■ Do *not* insert anything in the mouth (as tongue-biting occurs at seizure onset and cannot be prevented by observers)
■ If the convulsions continue for more than 5 minutes or recur without the person regaining consciousness, summon urgent medical attention
■ The person may be drowsy and confused for some 30–60 minutes and should not be left alone until fully recovered

Source: Allen et al. (1998)

2 years. Only 5% of children will continue to have convulsions into adult life.

Diagnosis

The diagnosis of epilepsy is essentially clinical. A detailed history from the patient can be reinforced by the accounts of eye witnesses. The key diagnostic features are shown in Table 4.

The main differential diagnosis of epilepsy is syncope. The latter is usually postural, is associated with prodromal symptoms and a very brief loss of consciousness and is rarely accompanied by after-effects.

Clinical examination is usually normal, but particular attention should be paid to the neurological and cardiovascular systems.

An abnormal EEG can confirm the clinical diagnosis and establish the type of epilepsy. Forty to fifty per cent of patients with epilepsy have a normal EEG between attacks. Further investigations are indicated if there is suspicion of non-idiopathic epilepsy (for example blood urea, glucose or calcium level) or an underlying structural cause (for example skull X-ray, computed tomography or magnetic resonance imaging).

Management

The immediate care of a person having a seizure involves first aid and common-sense measures to prevent injury (Table 5; Fig. 2). Once the diagnosis has been established (which usually involves referral to a neurologist), management entails the prevention of further fits, support and advice on issues relating to driving, employment and leisure activities.

Drug treatment is rarely started after a single fit – most neurologists will wait to see whether further episodes occur before committing a patient to long-term treatment.

Good or total control of the seizures can be expected in about 80% of patients using a single drug in an adequate dosage. There are many different anticonvulsants, the choice depending on the type of seizure, the age of the patient, the possibility of pregnancy, interaction with other medication and the likelihood of its producing unacceptable side-effects. It is possible to monitor the blood level of some anticonvulsants to obtain optimal control of the fits with minimal side-effects.

The most common first-line drugs for generalised and partial seizures are sodium valproate, carbamazepine ethosuximide, clonazepam and phenytoin, more recently introduced drugs such as lamotrigine, topiramate, gabapentin, levetiracetam and vigabatrin being reserved for those who do not respond or who encounter intolerable side-effects.

A periodic review of the continuing need for treatment is necessary, and after a period of the complete control of fits (usually 2–4 years), a gradual withdrawal over 6–12 months can be considered. With partial seizures, however, lifelong medication is recommended. Some patients with longstanding and/or intractable fits can be helped by stereotactic surgery.

Patients with newly diagnosed epilepsy require advice on risks relating to dangerous machinery and occupations, swimming, cycling and driving. In the UK, patients with epilepsy are not permitted to hold a heavy goods or public service vehicle licence. Once diagnosed, a patient with epilepsy must surrender his or her driving licence and cannot resume driving unless free of all fits for at least 1 year or if he or she has only nocturnal fits for at least 3 years (Box 3).

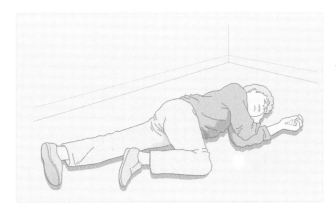

Fig. 2 **The adult recovery position.** This helps a semiconscious or unconscious person breathe and permits fluids to drain from the nose and throat. Note: not to be used if the person has a back or neck injury.

Epilepsy

- Epilepsy is a group of disorders rather than a disease.
- The majority of cases are idiopathic.
- A GP with 2000 patients may expect 1–2 new cases annually, 10–15 patients with epilepsy consulting and another 40–50 persons with a past history but no current problems.
- The fits can be generalised (grand mal, petit mal, akinetic or myoclonic) or partial (simple or complex)
- Diagnosis is essentially clinical but can be confirmed by an abnormal EEG.
- Management involves the prevention of further fits, support and advice on issues relating to driving, employment and leisure activities.
- 80% of patients with epilepsy can be well controlled on a single drug.

Migraine and other causes of recurrent headache

A sudden, severe headache occurring for the first time in any patient is always a potential worry as such an acute finding might well be serious. Meningitis is a particular worry, as is subarachnoid (brain) haemorrhage. It is important to stress that this section does not deal with these serious acute types of headache; it deals instead with subsequent episodes of headache that the patient and/or doctor recognise as (usually) being of the same kind. Paradoxically, it is normally the case that the longer that a patient has suffered episodes of severe headache, the *less likely they are to have a serious cause*.

There will be few if any readers who have not experienced a headache at some time in their lives. Headaches, like symptoms such as indigestion or muscle pain, are accepted by most people as a part of life so long as they do not occur too often or last too long, and especially when there is a fairly obvious cause such as a lack of sleep, worry about examinations or an over-indulgence in alcohol the night before!

Patients presenting with headache

When a patient consults a doctor about his or her headaches, that in itself is a significant piece of information: it means that the patient does not think that the headaches lie in the 'normal' range. Headache can be associated with a very large number of very different causes (Box 1), most of which are common and not a serious threat to health, although a few are seriously life-threatening.

Patients who regularly suffer from headaches come to recognise 'their' kind of headache and generally treat themselves by taking over-the-counter headache remedies and/or trying to avoid precipitating factors. Patients who do not usually suffer from headaches might be more liable to consult a doctor because they are aware that there are serious causes such as meningitis and brain tumours. A common misconception is that headaches are a sign of high blood pressure, but this is generally not true (as high blood pressure, at least initially, usually causes no symptoms). Parents are especially likely to suspect a brain tumour as a cause of headache in their children. However, even severe

---

Box 1 Causes of headache

Common
- Tension headache
- Headache secondary to infectious disease
- Migraine
- Referred pain from, for example, the sinuses, cervical spine, teeth, temporomandibular joints and eyes

Uncommon
- Head injury
- Drug-induced headache
- Neuralgia, for example herpetic or trigeminal
- Temporal arteritis

Rare/very rare
- Drug-induced headache
- Subarachnoid haemorrhage
- Brain tumour
- Cluster headache

---

headaches in children are very much more commonly caused by migraine (Box 2). A GP is unlikely to see even one patient with a headache arising from brain tumour in the whole of a professional lifetime.

We have chosen to write about headache and migraine principally because they are common phenomena that students can understand at an early stage of training. They provide a

good example of how doctors set about differentiating the cause of a symptom, in this case headache, and illustrate some of the principles of diagnosis that were outlined in pp 18–19.

Diagnosis

Although migraine is a very distinctive kind of headache with diagnostic features that have long been recognised in medical diagnosis, the mechanism by which it occurs is still uncertain. There have been shown to be temporary disturbances of blood flow in the brain, but this may be an effect of other underlying causes, such as changes in the level of important chemicals within the brain known as neurotransmitters. One called 5-hydroxytryptamine (5-HT) is currently thought to be important in the causation of migraine, partly because it has been found that medicines which affect 5-HT levels often relieve the headache.

The differentiating features of headaches are based mainly on the recognition of patterns that have been built up, partly by cumulative experience of the medical profession over a long period of time and partly by scientific investigation. Like much of medicine, this is a blend of 'art' and 'science'. Box 1 illustrates the many possible causes of headache.

Box 2 Headaches in children

Contrary to what used to be thought, children do suffer quite frequently from headache, but younger children may not identify or describe the symptom accurately. Older children can usually describe headaches quite well. Tension headache is probably much less common in children than in adults, but it can still occur, and children may also become depressed with associated headaches. It is important to enquire about possible difficulties at school or at home, and to ask the parents about emotional outbursts or behavioural disturbances, e.g. eating and sleeping problems, or problems with bowel or bladder control. As with adults, headache may (extremely rarely) be a symptom of increased intracranial pressure due, for example, to brain tumour. In that case, it is likely that other neurological symptoms, particularly unsteadiness of balance and gait, would be more prominent. Headaches from raised intracranial pressure classically take place in the early hours of the morning and are associated with vomiting; these symptoms wearing off as the morning progresses. The commonest cause of recurrent headache in children is migraine, with features similar to those in the adult. One main difference is that younger children more frequently complain of so-called 'migraine equivalents'. These kind of symptoms consist of cyclical attacks of vomiting, with or without abdominal pains and headache, which were formerly known as the 'periodic syndrome'. Frequently, as age increases, these children develop more classical migraine headache.

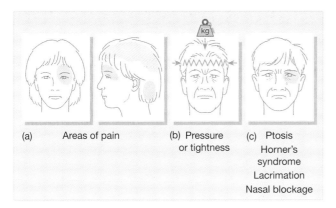

(a) Areas of pain   (b) Pressure or tightness   (c) Ptosis
Horner's syndrome
Lacrimation
Nasal blockage

Fig. 1 **'Safe' but unpleasant headaches. (a)** Migraine; **(b)** tension headache; **(c)** cluster headache.

Migraine

Migraine usually starts in adolescence and is more common and more severe in women. Patients come to recognise a variety of 'trigger factors' that bring on the attacks (Table 1). Box 3 shows how the classical features of a migraine attack can be *positively* identified.

Although there are other variants of migraine, there is before the headache starts classically some disturbance of vision: an inability to see clearly in part of the field of vision, for example, a misty, shimmering effect or, more dramatically, flashing lights. This tends to get progressively worse over about 15 minutes before the headache starts.

As the headache begins, the visual disturbance wears off. The headache is usually one sided, at least to start with, but may start on or spread to both sides. It usually gets progressively worse and is aggravated by stooping, exercise of any kind and particularly bright light. The nose may feel stuffy and congested, and the eyes may water. The patient usually feels sick and may actually vomit. Most patients learn to lie down and rest in a darkened room. In most cases, the symptoms pass off after a few hours sleep.

Most migraine sufferers do not have, however, the classical visual effects (or 'aura'), Box 2 referring to that more typical situation in which the diagnosis is slightly more difficult. If all or most of these features are present, a doctor can be fairly confident that the patient has migraine.

There are some fairly simple pointers that help to establish that the headaches are not likely to have a more serious cause, such as a brain tumour. Most important is the early age of onset. If an older person who had previously never suffered from headaches started to have them regularly, this might be an indication for the doctor to investigate more deeply. If these headaches were fairly recent in onset – i.e. the history were short – and were becoming progressively more frequent and/or more severe, this would provide a reason to investigate even more urgently.

These are of course only some illustrations of the more simple differentiating features. On the other hand, some differentiating features are more subtle and arise from medical and anatomical knowledge. For example, a vascular tumour of the brain (angioma) may very rarely mimic migraine. In this case, one of the main differentiating features is that the visual symptoms always occur on the same side (for anatomical reasons, the side opposite the tumour), whereas in migraine, the visual effects may affect opposite sides in different attacks, quite at random.

Cluster headaches ('migrainous neuralgia')

Although some of their features are similar, cluster headaches are quite distinct from migraine. In fact, they tend to occur in people who are not migraine sufferers, usually young men. There is often an excruciatingly severe pain, centred around one eye, with severe watering of the eye and blocking up of the nostril on the affected side at the peak of the attack. The severe pain usually subsides within about 1 hour, but the attacks may re-occur several times a day for a period of 4–6 weeks or even longer. Unlike migraine, the attacks are quite common during the night, disturbing sleep. After a pain-free period of several months, another cluster of headaches may occur. The condition is very disabling and is thought to be related to disturbance of the brain hormone serotonin.

Psychological causes

By far the most common cause of headaches is, however, simple tension and stress of various sorts, but otherwise unexplained headaches are also a feature of severe depression, which may not always be obvious from the demeanour of the patient. For example, some patients with depression 'put on a brave face' and may not admit to (or recognise) that they are depressed.

Table 1 **Common trigger factors for migraine**

- Stress and worry
- Missed meals
- Lack of sleep
- Stage of the menstrual cycle (usually pre-menstrual)
- Particular foodstuffs, e.g. chocolate, red wine and citrus fruits
- Caffeine withdrawal

Box 3 **Diagnostic criteria for migraine without aura**

- Attacks lasting 2–72 hours
- At least two of these features of the pain:
  - unilateral
  - pulsating
  - moderate to severe
  - aggravated by movement
- At least one of these associated features:
  - nausea
  - aggravated by light
  - aggravated by noise

To fulfil the full diagnostic criteria of the Classification Committee of the International Headache Society (1988), the patient must have had at least five attacks and have no other medical problem

---

Migraine and other recurrent headaches

- A severe, sudden headache occurring for the first time in any patient might be due to a serious cause, such as meningitis or brain haemorrhage, and needs urgent diagnosis and treatment.

- However, this section deals with recurrent headaches (usually where an initial diagnosis has previously been made), which might be severe, but are due to causes that are not usually life threatening.

- Many people have 'normal' headaches due to stress and lifestyle factors of various sorts. These 'tension headaches' may nonetheless be severe and troublesome.

- Migraine is a particular kind of common recurrent headache, the origin of which is still uncertain.

- Migrainous neuralgia is a much rarer variant.

- Usually these different kinds of headache can be positively distinguished from other conditions because they each have distinctive features.

Common gastrointestinal disorders

About 1 person in 10 consults the GP with a gastrointestinal disorder. Much chronic gastrointestinal disease is managed in general practice or by care shared between the GP and the hospital. About 1 person in 20 attending hospital does so because of GIT disease, which is low compared with 1 in 5 for cardiac disease. Managing such disease is expensive in terms of drugs and workload. In any general practice prescribing budget, the cost of histamine-2 (H_2) antagonists and proton pump inhibitors is a major item of expenditure.

Irritable bowel syndrome

Surveys of the prevalence of irritable bowel syndrome (IBS) in the general population suggest that between 15% and 25% of adults experience symptoms compatible with IBS in any 12 month period (Table 1). Those who consult their GP are in more distress, have more anxiety and depression, and suffer from more stressful life events than those who do not consult. Slightly more women than men suffer from the IBS, and slightly more women consult than men.

The history and physical examination of IBS are an important part of its management. Undergraduates are reluctant to make a diagnosis of IBS and tend to underestimate the distress it causes; patients may have hidden fears about their symptoms and may be puzzled at their recurrence. Reassurance and advice about increasing dietary fibre and fluid intake are an important part of management. A follow-up study at 1 year of 50 patients diagnosed with IBS indicated that 6 were free of symptoms, 18 had improved, but 25 showed no improvement and 1 was worse.

Gastro-oesophageal reflux disease

This is a chronic relapsing condition affecting 4–10% of the population. The

Table 1 Symptom complex of irritable bowel syndrome

- Abdominal pain
- Bowel disturbance (urgency and incontinence)
- Mucus
- A sensation of incomplete evacuation
- Distension
- Wind

Table 2 Symptom complex of gastro-oesophageal reflux disease

- Heartburn
- Bloating
- Epigastric tenderness
- Regurgitation
- Water brash (?)
- Severe pain
- Cough

symptom complex is described in Table 2.

Management

Patients with mild disease may be managed conservatively by raising the foot of the bed, taking antacids and adopting dietary discretion. Many will, however, need temporary or perhaps permanent acid suppression for symptom relief. H_2-receptor antagonists and proton pump inhibitors are the drugs of choice. Surgery is occasionally indicated where medication has failed. Fundoplication – buttressing of the gastro-oesophageal junction – is now the operation most commonly used to relieve this condition.

Patients with an endoscopic diagnosis of mild-to-moderate gastro-oesophageal reflux disease were followed up for 10 years: 70% still had their symptoms, 20% requiring daily acid suppression.

Peptic ulceration

Peptic ulceration has long been recognised as a product of self digestion. It results from an excess of autopeptic power of the gastric juices over the defences of the gastric and intestinal mucosa. At autopsy, 10% of women and 20% of men will have evidence of having had peptic ulceration. In Europe, duodenal ulceration is 2–4 times more common than gastric.

The natural history of peptic ulceration is difficult to predict, but a number of predisposing factors influence the incidence of frequent relapses and poor response to treatment (Table 3). Deep, large or multiple ulcers are more difficult to treat and are likely to relapse. Those patients with a high acid output are also more likely to have recurring illness, as are those who smoke and those with a family history of peptic

Table 3 Factors predisposing to peptic ulceration

- The role of diet is unclear – increased acid output may be involved, especially in duodenal ulceration
- Smoking
- *Helicobacter pylori* infection
- Corticosteroids
- Non-steroidal anti-inflammatory drugs
- Aspirin
- Family history
- Blood group O for duodenal ulcer

ulcer disease. Starting ulcer symptoms at a young age is a predictor of poor outcome.

Management is based around improving the mucosal defences and reducing acid secretion, using H_2-antagonists and proton pump inhibitors.

In one of the most remarkable changes in modern medicine, there has been a marked decline in the use of surgery for peptic ulceration: surgery is now reserved for intractable ulcers and has become a rare event.

Helicobactor pylori infection

Helicobactor pylori is one of the commonest human bacterial pathogens but was only discovered in 1984. The infection is related to increasing age and deprivation and is likely to be spread to other family members via the gastro-oral route. It initially produces an acute inflammatory gastritis and 15% of infected individuals develop a peptic ulcer. *H. pylori* increases the risk of gastric cancer in the long term. It produces urea, which is excreted in the breath and for diagnosis a breath testing kit has been developed which has high levels of sensitivity and specificity in referred populations. However, this may not be as good in primary care where the prior probability of disease is lower than in hospital.

The only evidence based indications for the treatment of *H. pylori* are for patients with duodenal or gastric ulcers. Eradication of the bacteria in patients with gastro-oesophageal reflux disease is highly contentious. Current treatment is by triple therapy which includes a proton pump inhibitor, clarithromycin, amoxycillin or metronidzole. Quadruple therapy is sometimes needed with the addition of bismuth.

The discovery that *H. pylori* is a cause of peptic ulcer has caused a significant reduction in the interest of psychological factors in peptic ulcer disease. However, there is good evidence that psychological factors trigger ulcers and it is reasonable to assume that stress, together with deprivation and increasing age, are all important co-factors with helicobactor in the aetiology of peptic disease.

Inflammatory bowel disease

The major inflammatory bowel diseases are ulcerative colitis and Crohn's disease. Over six new cases of each disease occur per 100 000 population per annum. A GP will see on average one new case of either ulcerative colitis or Crohn's disease each year.

Ulcerative colitis

This is more common in women. An environmental factor has been suggested in its aetiology by the observation that it is more common in US and Israeli Jews. There is a bimodal distribution, occurrences being seen in the 20–40 and 60–80-age groups. It occurs 15 times more commonly in first-degree relatives than in the general population (Table 4). Relapses are associated with outbreaks of gastroenteritis. Non-smokers are more prone than smokers to ulcerative colitis, and it is five times more common in Mormons.

Table 4 **Clinical feature of ulcerative colitis**	
Proctitis	25%
Left-sided colitis	50%
Total colitis	25%

The management of ulcerative colitis is symptomatic, corticosteroids being used either rectally or systemically in the acute attack. Maintenance treatment is with sulfasalazine derivatives. Immunosuppression with azathiaprine or ciclosporin is used in severe attacks, and anti-diarrhoeal agents are often needed. Surgery has a role, especially for abscesses, adhesions and severe unremitting disease. The risk of cancer is cumulative, with an incidence of 60% after 30 years with the disease.

Crohn's disease

Crohn's disease differs from ulcerative colitis in that it may affect any part of the gastrointestinal tract from the lips to the anus, the ileocolonic region being most commonly affected (Table 5). There are many extra-intestinal manifestations of Crohn's disease (Fig. 1).

Crohn's disease is most common in North America and Europe, is seen more in females than in males and has a unimodal distribution in the 15–40 age group. Seventeen per cent of patients with the condition have a positive family history. It is associated with ankylosing spondylitis, atopy and a high consumption of carbohydrates. In addition, it is three times more frequent in smokers.

The management of Crohn's disease is complex and involves managing the inflammatory process with steroids and immunosuppressants, correcting nutritional deficiencies and treating extra-intestinal manifestations. Some patients with Crohn's disease face a lifetime of surgery if medical treatment has failed, with intestinal obstruction, malabsorption, chronic blood loss and abscesses.

Data on the prognosis of Crohn's disease are based on hospital patients, which may give a rather less optimistic outlook. Managing the complications and maintaining a good nutritional status are however, important markers for a good outcome.

Coeliac disease

Coeliac disease is a bowel disorder resulting from a sensitivity to gluten, and similar proteins found in wheat, rye, oats and barley. It has classically been associated with diarrhoea and 'failure to thrive' in childhood but it can, in fact, present at any age with a wide variety of symptoms. These include fatigue, altered bowel habit, bloating, abdominal distension, depression and symptoms relating to iron deficiency anaemia and reduced vitamin B12 levels. Specific antibody

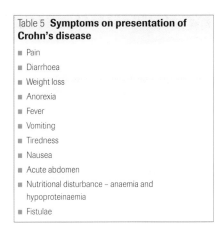

Table 5 **Symptoms on presentation of Crohn's disease**
■ Pain
■ Diarrhoea
■ Weight loss
■ Anorexia
■ Fever
■ Vomiting
■ Tiredness
■ Nausea
■ Acute abdomen
■ Nutritional disturbance – anaemia and hypoproteinaemia
■ Fistulae

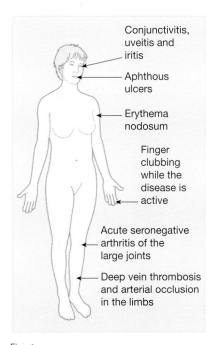

Fig. 1 **Crohn's disease with its many extra-intestinal manifestations.**

tests are now available, including AMA and TTG antibody levels, although the diagnosis is still made by taking D2 biopsies at OGD. The treatment is life-long adherence to a gluten free diet. This is quite complex and many patients find it difficult to adhere to this diet. The Coeliac Society (www.coeliac.org) offers excellent patient education and dietary information, and many gluten-free products are available on NHS prescription.

Common gastrointestinal disorders

■ H_2-antagonists and proton pump inhibitors are a major item of drug expenditure in general practice.

■ The prevalence of and distress caused by irritable bowel syndrome is often underestimated.

■ Deprivation and increasing age are all co-factors with *H. pylori* in the aetiology of peptic ulcer disease.

■ A GP will see a new case of Crohn's or ulcerative colitis once a year.

Prescribing/medicines utilisation

Please see Appendix 4 (p. 102) for an example of a UK prescription

In the UK as a whole, about 20% of all medicine consumed by the public is bought 'over the counter' (OTC) – without a doctor's prescription – the remainder being provided mostly on prescription through the NHS. Similarly, about 20% of all NHS medicines are provided through hospitals, the remaining 80% being prescribed in primary care. In 1997/98, about £8 billion was spent on medicines in the UK – roughly £150 per person, £115 per person being provided through the NHS. Nevertheless, in comparison with other countries, UK medicines consumption is moderate (Fig. 1), and the NHS is good value for money, costing about half as much as the mixed American-type public/private model.

As at January 2001, a charge of £6.20 is due for each NHS prescription item, but about 50% of patients are exempt from the charge (Table 1), and in 1996 only about 15% of items were charged for (because people who are exempt tend to receive most of the prescriptions).

Prescription of medicines

Although most medicines can be supplied on an NHS prescription, a written prescription from an authorised prescriber (doctor, dentist or, in limited circumstances, nurse prescriber) is a *legal requirement* only for those medicines classified as prescription-only medicines (POMs) by the licensing authority. Many medicines can be purchased directly

from a pharmacist (pharmacy, or P category) and some can be purchased from supermarkets and other general stores (general sale list, or GSL). Some POM medicines are specially tightly controlled (e.g. heroin, amphetamines and temazepam) mostly because of the potential for their abuse.

Many modern medicines are wonderfully effective. New treatments for stomach ulcer have, for example, virtually eliminated the need for major surgery, which was formerly the only effective treatment. Appendix 1 shows some of the commonly used drug groups and illustrates the important fact that they almost always have some bad, as well as good, effects. Even herbal remedies, which are generally thought to be harmless, can have adverse effects. St John's Wort, a plant extract taken for mild depression and as a 'pick me up', has, for example, been found to interfere with the effects of prescribed medicines such as warfarin and the contraceptive pill.

There are probably well over 1000 prescription medicines, most GPs limiting their use to a few hundred 'favourite' preparations so that they get

to know these well. There is a great deal of information support available to prescribers (Table 2) – in some ways too much. In the UK the National Institute of Clinical Excellence (NICE), set up in 1999, will help by disseminating authoritative national guidance. Computerised decision support systems (such as PRODIGY, a system widely used in general practice in England), which selectively present evidence-based information to help the prescriber to choose the best medicine(s) for a particular individual patient, will become increasingly sophisticated and an essential tool for handling the information overload.

Increasingly, other health professionals are involved in prescribing in primary care. Some nurses can already prescribe in a limited way, and a recent government review will considerably extend this in future. Pharmacists in particular have an important role in helping GPs to maintain high-quality prescribing (see Table 3).

Proprietary (brand) and generic names

Most drugs are known by both brand and generic names. The generic name is an officially approved name for all preparations of that drug: propranolol, for example, is the generic name for a medicine commonly used in the treatment of heart disease and high

---

Table 1 Exemption from prescription charges in NHS

- Children under 16 years of age and some students
- Those aged over 60
- Those carrying a health authority exemption (maternity) certificate
- Sufferers of some chronic illnesses, e.g. diabetes, hypothyroidism and epilepsy
- War pensioners
- Those on a low income
- Oral contraceptives (provided free to all)

Table 2 Examples of information support available to prescribers

- General journals – e.g. *British Medical Journal* and *British Journal of General Practice*
- Specific journals and periodicals – e.g. *Prescribers' Journal, Drug and Therapeutics Bulletin, National Prescribing Centre MeRec Bulletins, Prescriber and Medicines Resource* (Scotland)
- Formularies – principally the British National Formulary, which is now also available in CD-ROM form. Most regions also have local formularies constructed around the British National Formulary

---

Table 3 Ways in which pharmacists can provide prescribing support for GPs

- Monitoring drug therapy for individual patients, e.g. reviewing repeat prescriptions
- Services to nursing and residential homes, by auditing prescribing for residents
- Prescribing analysis, reviewing general treatment policies, using PACT or SPA data
- Formulary development
- Discharge prescribing and liaison with hospitals

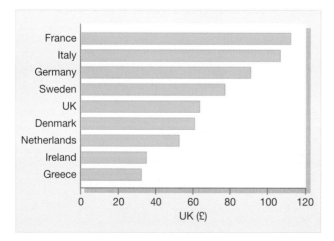

Fig. 1 **Histogram showing cost of all medicines taken per person per year (1990).** The UK cost is about 23% below the average for Europe and 40% less than that in the USA.

Table 4 **The more commonly prescribed groups of medicines by GPs (1992)**		
Medicines for treatment of:	Percentage of all prescriptions	Percentage of total cost
Nervous system (includes some pain-killers as well as e.g. antidepressants and sedatives)	18	11
Heart and circulation	17	19
Infections	11	7
Respiratory conditions (e.g. asthma)	10	12
Stomach and gut	8	14
Skin	7	5
Muscles and joints	6	8
Endocrine system (e.g. diabetes)	5	7

Source: House of Commons Health Committee (1994)

blood pressure, which is marketed diversely under five different brand names in the UK, and under additional names in different countries.

The only difference between brands is in general the price, unbranded preparations, paracetamol BP rather than the common brand-named Panadol, for example, being cheaper. For clarity, lack of confusion and economy, it is usually best to prescribe by generic name. Most computer systems can do this automatically.

Control and licensing of medicines
In the UK, medicines have to be licensed by the Minister of Health through the Medicines Control Agency before they can be put into general use. There is a strict control over the safety and effectiveness of medicines, monitored by the Medicines Control Agency and the Committee on Safety of Medicines, which is the main government advisory body. The licensing authorities are not, however, legally allowed to consider comparative efficacy or comparative cost (i.e. how well a new medicine works or how much it costs compared with existing treatments). A new medicine might therefore have to be licensed even if it costs more and is less effective than an existing treatment, so long as it has been proved to be safe and to work

better than a placebo (inactive) preparation for the illness in question. Drug licensing will increasingly be carried out across the European Union as a whole rather than separately in the constituent countries, being co-ordinated by the European Medicines Evaluation Agency.

Monitoring medicines
Any unwanted detrimental effects of medicines (adverse drug reactions) often do not become obvious until the medicine is widely used. Drug companies must tell the Medicines Control Agency of any adverse reactions reported to them, and all prescribers and pharmacists are also encouraged to send their findings to the Committee on Safety of Medicines, especially if the medication has been licensed for less than 2 years. These medicines are identified by a black triangle (▼) in all the literature, and they should be used with special care.

Repeat prescribing
Long-term treatment for chronic diseases such as asthma, high blood pressure, heart disease, arthritis, thyroid disorders and diabetes dominates prescribing in general practice. Many patients with these conditions need routine medical review perhaps annually or 6-monthly, but they require a more frequent

renewal of their regular prescriptions because it is generally not desirable to provide a 6 or 12 months supply of medication all at once. About 75% of all GP prescriptions are 'repeats' – the same prescription being issued at (usually monthly) intervals to make sure that the patient has an adequate regular supply without having too great a 'hoard'.

Some of these prescriptions are issued by the doctor when the patient coincidentally consults for some other reason, but most are issued by GP computer systems at the patient's request, without seeing the doctor. A well set-up system should check that the patient is requesting medicines at the right intervals and alert the patient and doctor when a medical review is needed.

Prescribing analyses and cost
The pharmacist dispenses the patient's prescription and then sends it to the Prescription Pricing Authority for payment. The authority collects presenting analysis and cost (PACT) data on all prescriptions throughout the country and feeds back to all practices regular summaries of what has been prescribed. These data are of limited value, but practices can use them as the starting point for an analysis of prescribing habits. The Prescription Pricing Authority data have been widely used to examine variations in prescribing, for example between practices or geographical regions. Some variation is caused by a difference in doctors' prescribing habits, but most is generally considered to be the result of a genuine difference in illness rates in different populations. The Information Services Division (ISD) and the Scottish prescribing analysis (SPA) comprise the Scottish equivalent of this system.

Prescribing/medicines utilisation

- In the UK about a fifth of all medicines are purchased directly without a prescription.

- UK medicines consumption is moderate in comparison with many other countries.

- Increasingly, in UK and elsewhere, health professionals other than doctors (e.g. nurses, pharmacists, chiropodists) are, or will be, legally able to prescribe some medicines.

- Like most governments, the UK carefully controls medicines production through licensing of medicines.

- In the NHS, government agencies also increasingly try to influence and monitor how medicines are used.

The hospital – general practice interface

As described on page 8, there are considerable similarities between different countries in the clinical problems presenting in primary care and in terms of health indices such as infant mortality, birth and fertility rates and life expectancy. There are, however, marked differences in the total health expenditure between these countries. This is largely explained by differences in their administrative and funding systems, a key component of which is the primary–secondary care interface.

In all countries, hospital-based services account for the majority of health services expenditure – 60% of the total in the UK. The 'gatekeeper' role of the GP, described on pages 2–3, has probably contributed to the UK's comparatively lower level of expenditure compared with that of other countries. Indeed, it has been shown that a higher primary care orientation of a health-care system is likely to produce better health of a population at lower costs (Starfield 1992).

Workload

Because of the selection of patients through the referral process, the hospital specialist encounters a totally different range of problems from those of the GP. Broadly speaking, specialists tend to see rare diseases or atypical versions of common diseases. Figure 1 shows a graphic representation of this difference.

The traditional and most common interface between primary and secondary care is via the referral of patients by GPs to hospital specialists, as either inpatients or outpatients. Although 90% of episodes of illness presenting to GPs are dealt with in primary care, 18% of the population are newly referred to a specialist each year. This accounts for 25% of outpatient activity. GPs make on average about five outpatient referrals per 100 consultations (12 referrals per 100 registered patients) per year. There is a considerable variation (threefold or fourfold) between individual practitioners and between practices (Wilkin 1992). The main reason for referring patients to specialist outpatient clinics are shown in Table 1.

The primary–secondary care interface is, however, dynamic and constantly changing. Demographic and political changes, coupled with technological developments and ongoing health reforms, have all contributed to a radical change in the way in which GPs and hospital specialists relate and interact.

Table 1 Reasons for referral

- Diagnosis
- Investigation
- Advice on treatment
- Specialist treatment
- A second opinion
- Reassurance for the patient
- Sharing the load, or risk, of treating a difficult or demanding patient
- A deterioration in the GP–patient relationship, leading to a desire to involve someone else in managing the problem
- A fear of litigation
- Direct requests by patients or relatives

Source: Coulter (1998)

The changing interface

There has, in general, been a trend for more secondary care services to transfer to the community. There also has been a resurgence of interest in community hospitals, which tend to be situated in more rural areas, offer low-tech services and be run by GPs with specialist back-up as required. In the USA and Canada, many family doctors (the equivalent of GPs) have admitting privileges and provide inpatient care for their patients. This is not the case in UK, although over one quarter of GPs have clinical assistant posts in hospital specialities such as dermatology, ENT, gastroenterology and geriatric medicine. Such posts have provided a practical method of increasing GPs' expertise in particular clinical areas. A recent innovation is the introduction of GPs with Special Interests (see p. 13).

Diversity of models

Many different models of delivering clinical care traverse the primary–secondary care interface. A selection (not necessarily comprehensive) of these is shown in Table 2.

Shared care

This term covers a wide range of activities, formerly the exclusive domain of the hospital specialist. The responsibility for the care of the patient is shared between the hospital staff and the GP, practice teams and community health staff. Shared care was pioneered with antenatal patients but particularly lends itself to the management and monitoring of chronic diseases such as diabetes and asthma. Shared care is most common in the outpatient setting

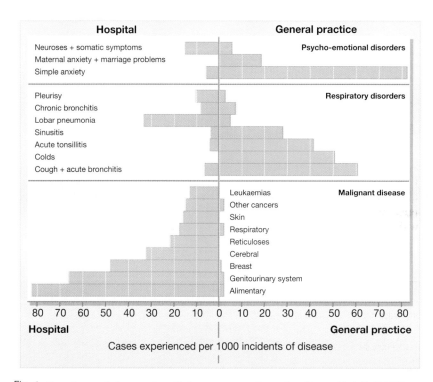

Fig. 1 **Experience of disease: hospital versus general practice.** Source: Hodgkin (1985.)

Table 2 **Models of delivering care across the primary–secondary care interface**
■ Shared care
■ Outreach clinics
■ Hospital-at-home
■ Managed care

Table 3 **Factors contributing towards effective shared care**
■ Patient co-operation or shared care cards
■ Initial and continuing GP education
■ Written treatment and management protocols
■ An effective patient record and recall system
■ Protected GP time to perform the necessary duties
■ Effective communication
■ The appointment of a liaison officer

Source: Hampson et al (1996)

Table 4 **Factors changing the hospital – GP interface**
■ Telemedicine
■ Remote diagnosis
■ Patient-held 'smartcards'
■ Internet and e-mail
■ Near-patient testing
■ Liaison nurses
■ Community specialists

but can be applied in the patient's home and in hospital.

The traditional model of outpatient care, centred in the hospital clinic, makes an efficient use of specialist time and allows easy access to other secondary care services. Getting to the hospital can, however, be difficult, expensive and time-consuming for patients. There can also be problems with communication, delay in treatment, duplication of effort, unnecessary procedures, long waiting lists, inappropriate follow-up and high cost (Orton 1994). A number of factors can contribute to effective shared care (Table 3).

With shared outpatient care, the patient usually still attends the specialist at hospital, but visits may be split between the hospital and the general practice surgery. Patient-held or shared-care cards facilitate communication. This model is now commonly used for patients with diabetes, asthma, HIV infection and some mental illnesses, and for those receiving antenatal or geriatric care.

Outreach clinics

This is a development of shared care in which hospital-based specialists provide diagnostic and treatment services in a primary care setting. A survey of hospital managers in England and Wales found that over half of all hospitals were providing one or more such clinics in a wide range of specialties (Bailey et al 1994). These clinics are sometimes merely a relocation from the hospital. More commonly, however, there is some form of liaison between the specialist and the GP, actual joint consultations sometimes occurring.

Outreach clinics have been

established over a wide range of specialties and areas from psychiatry to obstetrics, asthma to orthopaedics and care of the dying to dermatology.

Hospital-at-home schemes

These schemes bring high-tech, intensive procedures and skills from the hospital into patients' homes. Examples include haemodialysis and parenteral nutrition services.

Managed care

'Managed care' applies to a wide range of activities occurring in a variety of organisational settings, a helpful definition being:

> *a variety of methods of financing and organising the delivery of comprehensive health care in which an attempt is made to control costs by controlling the provision of services*
> (Inglehart 1993).

Managed care originated in the US but has evolved to influence health-care systems in many countries, including the UK, New Zealand, Spain and Italy.

The two main organisational settings for delivering managed care are the health maintenance organisation and the preferred providers organisation. There are three dimensions of managed care (Rosleff and Lister 1995):

■ health policy
■ systems management (how the policy is administered)
■ disease management (how diseases presenting to the system are dealt with).

The main aim of managed care is to cut cost while maintaining quality, but there is conflicting evidence of its success in achieving this.

Further developments (Table 4)

Telemedicine has meant that specialist opinion has become immediately accessible to the most isolated sites, and the remote interpretation of ECGs and ultrasound scans is readily available. Computer technology has enabled patients to carry 'smartcards' storing vital medical information, immediately available for any medical consultation in hospital or general practice. E-mail and the Internet have made a vast amount of medical information readily accessible to specialists, GPs – and patients.

Patient testing and the electronic delivery of test results are re-defining the role of the hospital laboratory and allowing GPs to take increasing responsibility for diagnosing, managing and monitoring diseases. Liaison nurses, specially trained as experts in particular areas such as asthma, terminal care, diabetes and stroke care, can provide information, services and support from their hospital bases to patients and primary care teams.

A new type of specialist – the community specialist – is evolving in response to these changes. Although based in hospital, these doctors provide a link between acute hospital services and care in the community; posts already exist in areas such as paediatrics, cardiology, respiratory medicine, psychiatry, diabetic medicine and geriatrics.

The hospital – GP interface

■ The 'gatekeeper' role of the GP is a critical factor in controlling access to secondary care and its associated expenditure.

■ 18% of the population are newly referred to a specialist each year.

■ The primary–secondary care interface is dynamic and constantly changing.

■ There has been a recent trend for secondary care services to transfer to the community.

■ Further changes are inevitable with advances in medical technology and information

Community care: a UK perspective

There are many definitions of community care, one of the simplest being that used by the UK Department of Health (Box 1). Over the past 20 years or so, there has been a steady move towards providing more care in the community. This development has been driven partly by philosophical, ideological and political trends and partly by a belief that costs might be cut or savings made (Fig. 1). There has been a major shift away from institutional care, particularly for older people, the mentally ill and those with physical and learning difficulties.

More recently, there has been a growing recognition that the special needs of many individuals and groups can be best met by providing community-based services. A list of such groups (by no means comprehensive) is shown in Box 2. The advantages of community care for these patients or clients are that services can be:

- easily accessible
- tailored to local needs

Box 1 Definition of community care

Community care means providing the service and support which people who are affected by problems of ageing, mental illness, mental handicap or physical or sensory disability need to be able to live as independently as possible in their homes, or in 'homely' settings in the community.

Source: Secretaries of State (1989)

Box 2 Groups of people for whom community care services are provided

- Children
- Older people
- Adolescents
- Pregnant women
- Those who are mentally ill
- Those with learning difficulties
- People with physical difficulties
- Those with a terminal illness
- The homeless
- Refugees
- Ethnic minorities
- People with alcohol and drug problems
- Those in specific disease groups, e.g. diabetics, HIV-positive people

Table 1 **Example of the spectrum of care settings for older people**	
Care at home	Personal care and practical help provided to older people in their own homes
Adult placement	Placing older people with selectively matched carers in the carer's own home
Day care	Includes NHS day hospitals and local authority and independent sector day centres
Sheltered housing	Individual housing within a setting that offers different degrees of monitoring, protection or support. It can be owned or rented. Within this there are the following variations: ■ very sheltered housing or housing with extra care ■ retirement communities/care villages
Residential care	Care for older people in an institutional setting, either in a residential or a nursing home
NHS continuing care	Nursing homes, hospices and community hospitals

Source: Royal Commission on Long Term Care (1999)

- geographically close
- provided by local professionals or care workers.

As the boundaries between primary and secondary care have become more blurred, community care has taken on increasing importance.

As community care has developed, many disciplines and health professionals have become involved, but nurses still constitute the majority of the workforce. The skills of these health professionals are augmented by those of the numerous voluntary workers and organisations operating in the community. There are hundreds of patient support groups, societies and charities that offer advice, information and services to patients and their carers; some examples are Age Concern, the British Diabetic Association and the Alzheimer's Society.

Care settings

Community care is provided in a range of settings by the public, private and voluntary sectors. There is a wide variation in practice and form within each, and an increasing overlap, as innovative approaches are developed. A typical spectrum for older people is summarised in Table 1.

Changing face of community care

Community care is undergoing a dynamic change as a result of several interrelated developments in our society:

1. demographic changes – an increase in the number of older people
2. major reforms of the health and social services, including the 1990 NHS and Community Care Act, which transferred the financial responsibility for residential and nursing home care from the social security budget to local authorities
3. devolution at both national and local government levels
4. technological developments such as telemedicine, electronic communication and assistive technology (purpose-designed devices or systems that enable people to perform tasks they otherwise could not)

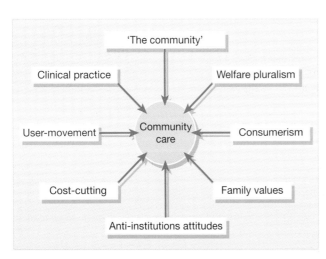

Fig. 1 **Influences on community care.** Source: Atkinson (1999)

5. an increasing involvement of the public, patients and carers in developing and planning services.

Although the development of a primary care-led or driven NHS has removed many of the barriers between primary and secondary care, there is still a considerable organisational divide between health and social services, between health authorities and local government. In 1999, the Royal Commission on Long Term Care drew the following conclusions:

- There needs to be more effective joint working and a greater sharing of responsibility between health, social services and housing authorities.
- There should be a greater emphasis on rehabilitation.
- There should be a more consistent framework for assessment and eligibility for long-term care.
- More opportunities should be available to enable people to stay at home.
- More support should be offered to carers.
- There should be more real choice offered.
- The services offered should be culturally sensitive.
- There should be a greater emphasis on quality.
- The system should be easier to access.
- A new relationship of trust between clients, carers and services must be created.

The expenditure on long-term care services was £11 billion in 1995 and is estimated to increase to £20 billion in 2020 and £45 billion in 2050. If, however, disability associated with ageing fell by 1% per year, the cost would, all else being equal, be reduced to £28 billion in 2050 (Royal Commission on Long Term Care 1999).

The notion of 'intermediate' care has been proposed as a solution to the recurrent problem of a shortage of acute hospital beds in the winter months. The number of beds per head of population for acute, general and maternity care has fallen by over 2% a year since 1980, despite a rise in the number of acute and general admissions per head of population of around 3.5% a year. Two-thirds of hospital beds are occupied by patients aged over 65, and half of the rapid increase in emergency admission in the past 5 years has been accounted

for by people aged over 75. Convalescent centres would build a bridge between home and hospital for older people and could be based in major hospitals, revitalised cottage or community hospitals, hospital-at-home systems or newly built units.

Saving Lives: Our Healthier Nation

This White Paper on public health (Secreatry of State for Health 1999), acknowledged that the social, economic and environmental factors tending to cause poor health are potent, and it proposed a partnership of people, communities and government working together to improve health. This broader approach, extending well beyond the limited medical model, will involve a range of initiatives on education, welfare-to-work, housing neighbourhoods, transport and the environment aimed at improving health rather than treating disease. Three particular initiatives that offer opportunities to develop community care by encouraging a partnership between local authorities and the NHS are:

1 Health Action Zones
2. Healthy Living Centres
3. Health Improvement Programmes.

Heath Action Zones are areas of England that have been granted special status and additional funding to tackle health inequalities and promote new ways of working together locally between health and social services. There are currently 26 such areas throughout the country, located in regions of health and social deprivation such as Tyne and Wear, inner city London, Wolverhampton and Merseyside.

Healthy Living Centres are resource centres where local people can access social and welfare services, exercise and leisure facilities, and advice on legal matters, nutrition, transport, home safety and housing, as well as

medical services. These centres are complementary to *Our Healthier Nation* and to the achievement of local health targets, and focus on health in its broadest sense, providing opportunities to improve the quality of life and to enable people to achieve their full potential.

Health Improvement Programmes are action programmes to improve health and health care locally, being led by the health authority. They involve NHS Trusts, primary care groups and other primary care professionals such as dentists, opticians and pharmacists working in partnership with the public and the local authority and engaging other local interests. Health Improvement Programmes (Secretary of State for Health 1997) will cover:

- the most important health needs of the local population and how these are to be met by the NHS and its partner organisations through a broader action on public health
- the main health-care requirements of local people and how local services should be developed to meet them, either directly by the NHS or, where appropriate, jointly with social services
- the range, location and investment required in local health services to meet the needs of local people.

Health Improvement Programmes will be the vehicles for implementing National Service Frameworks, which will:

- set national standards and define service models for a specific service or care group
- put in place programmes to support their implementation
- establish performance measures against which progress within an agreed timetable will be measured.

National Service Frameworks exist for diabetes, renal diseases, mental health and coronary heart disease (Secretary of State for Health 1999).

Community care: a UK perspective

- Community care means providing the right level of intervention and support to enable people to achieve maximum independence and control over their own lives.
- More care is being provided outside hospitals and institutions for a wider range of people or clients.
- Community care is provided in a range of settings, involving multi-disciplinary working and informal carers.
- The boundaries between health care and social care are becoming blurred, helped by initiatives such as Health Action Zones, Healthy Living Centres and Health Improvement Programmes.

Complementary and alternative medicine

Orthodox medicine generally claims to be founded on biomedical science, but its roots are not so far removed from the quackery of which complementary and alternative therapists are often accused. Indeed, it was mainly the fear of widespread quackery in conventional medicine in USA at the turn of the 20th century that led Abraham Flexner to devise the modern model of the university-based medical school, founded on the underlying disciplines of (mostly laboratory-based) medical science (Berliner 1985).

As a consequence, conventional medicine did indeed become, during the 20th century, increasingly based on scientific evidence but still, to an alarmingly limited extent, so that, even now in the 21st century, many treatments that are in routine use have little or no scientifically established basis. On the one hand, this has led to a drive for 'evidence-based practice', so it is increasingly difficult for conventional doctors to justify the use of even long-established and cherished treatments for which there is no scientific basis. On the other hand, there has also been an increasing recognition that rigorous scientific method has limitations in its application. We do not yet, for example, fully understand why, in rigorous scientific trials, patients with symptoms or diseases that are real and potentially serious may respond to 'placebo' (i.e. scientifically inactive) treatments.

This may in part explain the paradox that whereas conventional medicine is becoming increasingly 'scientific', patients and some doctors appear increasingly to be turning towards complementary and alternative therapies that frequently appear to have no possible basis in conventional science, even entering the realms of mysticism (Box 1).

Why do patients seek complementary and alternative therapies

The British Medical Association conducted a survey to identify why patients sought these therapies. The report was critical of CAM generally but identified four factors that appeared to be common to them and to attract patients:

Box 1 A framework for differentiating between disciplines

Complete systems of care
Diagnostic, investigative and therapeutic approaches that are different from those present in Western medicine:
- Osteopathy/chiropractic
- Acupuncture/traditional Chinese medicine
- Homeopathy
- Herbal medicine

Diagnostic methods
Ways of determining the presence or absence of disease:
- Iridology
- Kinesiology
- Hair analysis
- Aura diagnosis

Therapeutic procedures
Different approaches to treatment:
- Massage therapy
- Aromatherapy
- Spiritual healing
- Reflexology
- Hydrotherapy

Self-help approaches
Activities undertaken by patients individually or in groups:
- Meditation
- Breathing and relaxation
- Exercise – yoga and tai chi
- Nutritional, e.g. fasting or dieting

Table 1 Rise in public interest in complementary medicine

- An estimated 4–5 million people a year in the UK go to complementary practitioners
- Approximately 14–20% of patients with chronic disease have consulted a complementary practitioner
- About 75% of the public support NHS access to complementary medicine
- There is continuing public scepticism about drugs and their side-effects
- Media optimism and support for complementary therapies is being maintained
- There may be an increased public desire to take more responsibility for their health choices

- *Time* – the consultations were longer than those offered by doctors in the NHS.
- *Relationship* – the exchange and communication between therapist and patient was felt to be more 'equal'.
- *Touch* – many CAMs (osteopathy, massage etc) use touch.
- *Charisma* – the unknown and often esoteric language used by some therapists appeared to impress patients.

A more detailed survey by Ernst et al (1995) reported the following reasons:

1. because they want to use all possible options in health care – 57.8%
2. because they hope to be cured without side-effects – 47.9%
3. because it is their last hope – 37.9%
4. because they have previously had a good experience – 37.9%
5. because they are disappointed by orthodox medicine – 31.8%
6. because they feel that they will be better understood – 28.9%
7. because they are inclined towards unscientific ideas – 8.1%
8. because they are not really ill – 4.3%
9. because it usually costs more – 3.8%.

Other surveys indicate fewer positive reasons why some patients seek CAM, but some of these findings may also reflect the opinions of the researchers that:

- patients may be are psychologically less stable
- the wealthy 'worried well' are

attracted to such treatment

- the population is naïve, optimistic and gullible
- there is a distrust of scientific explanations.

There is also a view that 'market forces' and choice, together with a consumerist approach to health care, encourage many patients to 'try something different'.

What conditions are treated by CAM?

Most patients seek CAM directly, although there is an increasing number of examples of co-operative approaches between CAM and orthodox medicine. Some GPs employ therapists directly to work alongside them, whereas some refer to a selected group. Pain clinics and anaesthetists occasionally make use of acupuncture as an additional approach to the management of difficult cases.

Most surveys suggest that the most often quoted reason for seeking CAM is for the 'relief of symptoms', these symptoms falling into two distinct groupings – pain (from musculosketal disorders such as arthritis, trauma and back pain) and psychological distress (anxiety, depression and stress insomnia). Notwithstanding these surveys, the largest group of therapists in the UK are spiritual healers, which suggests that orthodox medicine, with its emphasis on science and a high-tech approach, does not offer what some patients seek and identify that they need.

Research evidence for the efficacy and safety of CAM

There have been several obstacles for research studies in CAM. These include a lack of funding, a lack of research skills, a lack of academic interest and a lack of patients. Also, there is a deep and continuing conceptual conflict with regard to research methodologies. The supporters of CAM largely reject randomised controlled trials as an instrument to measure efficacy,

Table 2 Clinical trial evidence in complementary medicine – conclusions from recent, authoritative systemic reviews and meta-analyses

	Acupuncture	Homeopathy	Manipulation
Conditions	Chronic pain	Any	Low back pain
Type of data summarised	14 RCTs of various acupuncture treatments	89 randomised and/or controlled trials	8 RCTs of chiropractic
Method of evaluation	Systematic review	Meta-analysis	Systematic review
Conclusion	'Various sources of bias, including problems with blindness, precluded a conclusive finding'	'Clinical effects of homeopathy [not] completely due to placebo'	'[No] convincing evidence for the effectiveness of chiropractic for acute or chronic low back pain'.

RCT, randomized controlled trial
Data from Patel et al (1989), Linde et al (1997) and Assendelft et al (1996)

whereas orthodox doctors will only accept studies that conform to traditional scientific enquiry. Although this debate is still continuing, there is nevertheless an increasing literature on CAM, most of it revealing few or no positive results (Table 2). However, many herbal medicines have been shown to work in conventional scientific trials, for example, St John's Wort for mild depression, ginko biloba for dementia and palmetto for the urinary obstruction caused by (non-cancerous) enlargement of the male prostate gland (Ernst 2000).

It seems likely that, in general, most CAM methods are, at least, not likely to be harmful and serious adverse effects seem to be rare, especially with physical methods. However, Chinese herbal remedies in particular have recently been associated with serious illness and several deaths across Europe, mainly from bad effects on the liver and kidneys. In general, there may be a public misperception that herbal and plant substances are safe because they are 'natural'. However, many 'natural' substances are potentially lethal to humans, particularly if too much is taken. Many powerful orthodox medicines were originally derived from plants or moulds (e.g. digoxin, opiates and penicillin) in carefully standardised doses. In contrast, the contents and potency of herbal medicines may vary greatly and they are not subject to the strict regulation applying to pharmaceuticals, although many experts think they should be.

Bad effects may also arise if people rely entirely on CAM and avoid orthodox medicine altogether. There have been a few examples of serious illness or death resulting from people not seeking orthodox medical treatment that would have been effective, either for themselves or their children. The extent of lesser but still important instances of ill-health arising from this effect is unknown because it has not been adequately studied.

Conclusion

There is little or no scientific basis for most CAM, but that is not to say that these therapies have been proved to have no effect. By their very nature, they are difficult to test in a conventional scientific way. Some may have an apparent effect in individuals as a result of the ill-understood 'placebo effect'. Some (like acupuncture) may have a weak effect through hitherto unknown mechanisms.

It seems probable, however, that none of these CAM therapies has a major effect, particularly in the treatment of life-threatening or serious disease. Orthodox medicine offers the only hope for those with serious disease, and there is a danger that the more fanatical exponents of CAM might risk the health of their patients. Otherwise, provided that users accept its limitations, CAM may provide additional succour, particularly when conventional medicine has no answer.

Complementary and alternative medicine

- Increasing interest among the public, the medical profession and health-care planners has resulted in major development in CAM over the past 10 years

- There is little or no scientific basis for CAM but that is not to say that all CAM therapies have proved ineffective.

- Some may work via a 'placebo effect' and others may have a weak but real effect via unknown mechanisms.

- Most CAM is harmless, but some herbal medicines are unsafe.

Genetics in primary care

Primary care has, traditionally, had only a small part to play in genetic medicine. A GP might previously have become knowledgeable about a single gene disorder if it affected a family on his list, GPs were otherwise only very familiar with the importance of the impact of familial disease from a social and cultural viewpoint. The advent of the 'new genetics' has seen an increase in the importance of genetics in primary care consultations, especially in the field of hereditary cancers and screening. It is probable that the GP's role in this area will increase further, for example in the field of common diseases such as diabetes mellitus and hypertension, and particularly if genetic testing can predict an individual patient's response to a particular drug.

What is different about genetics?

There are two aspects of genetic medicine that set it apart from other branches of medicine. First, a person's genome is unalterable, so the diagnosis of a gene disorder is 'for life'. Interventions may be appropriate to lessen the impact of the mutation, but it will be a long time before gene therapy can correct the mutation. Second, a genetic diagnosis has implications not only for the patient, but also for his or her blood relatives. GPs rarely counsel patients for gene testing because such counselling is time-consuming and GPs are usually not in a position to contact other family members, because they care for nuclear rather than extended families.

The family history

The family history is used in four different ways in primary care:

1. It can help a GP to understand the social and cultural aspects of a patient's presenting problem. Family medicine involves a knowledge of the interaction between patients, their families and their environment. The impact of a disease in one person on another family member (a patient caring for a disabled relative becoming depressed, for example) or a patient's concern about developing a disease that has affected another family member, even if there is in fact no hereditary basis for it ('Could my headache be caused by a brain tumour because that is what my father died of?'). Diseases clustering in a family may be the result of a shared environment rather than hereditary factors.

2. The family history can be used as part of a risk assessment during history-taking. A doctor may have a lower threshold for undertaking investigations for heart disease in a patient with chest pain and a number of relatives who have suffered premature heart disease.

3. A formal family history (known as a 'pedigree', or a 'genogram' in USA) can be used to assess a patient worried about a disease known to have a hereditary basis.

4. The family history can be employed as a screening tool. Patients are often asked at registration or health checks whether there is any known family history of disease. This may be appropriate in some circumstances. Family history-taking does not, however, fulfil the criteria of a screening test as it cannot usually be followed up with a proven intervention.

Taking a family history

Taking a family history is the key skill in the assessment of any genetic problem. It requires practice to remember the key questions (Table 1),

the symbols to use (Fig. 1) and how to set the family history out on the page. The pedigree diagram is an excellent way of setting down family information succinctly and can form the basis of a referral letter to secondary care. It takes 10–15 minutes to take a family history over three generations, which usually requires a specially arranged extended consultation.

Interpretation of the family history requires a knowledge of the disease and its probable pattern of inheritance

Table 1 **Taking the family history**
■ Date the history
■ Identify the presenting patient (proband) with an arrow. Note the ethnic origin
■ Move across a generation (i.e. patient to siblings) and then move up or down to next generation
■ For those alive, record their sex, age/date of birth and medical history
■ For those who are dead, record the sex, age at death and cause of death
■ For significant illnesses, record the age at diagnosis. If you are interested in assessing one illness, concentrate on this and any related illnesses, e.g. breast and ovarian cancer
■ Aim for first- and second-degree relatives over three generations. This may need to be extended if a suspicious pattern develops
■ Ask about consanguinity (marriage between second cousins or closer relatives) as this is important in autosomal recessive disease
■ Ask specifically about children who have died, physically/mentally handicapped relatives, adoptions, miscarriages, still births and half-siblings

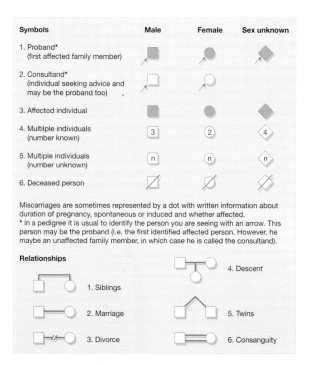

Fig. 1 **The symbols used in a pedigree.**

Box 1 Inherited cancers

Approximately 5% of breast, ovarian and colorectal cancers are inherited. Two dominantly inherited genes have already been identified for breast cancer (*BRCA1* and *BRCA2*) and two for colorectal cancer, causing familial adenomatous polyposis and hereditary non-polyposis colorectal cancer.

The GP's role in the management of patients presenting with a family history suggestive of an inheretied cancer is fourfold:

1. Identify those patients at high risk who may benefit from referral (Table 2).
2. Counsel these patients so that they have realistic expectations of a referral. Most patients are not high risk and will not be offered a genetic test. It is only practical to offer a genetic test to a patient if a gene mutation has been identified in an affected family member. There are a limited number of interventions for patients at high risk, for example mammography for breast cancer or colonoscopy for colorectal cancer, but neither of these interventions have been subjected to randomised controlled trials. The main advantage of genetic testing in patients at risk of inheriting a dominant gene is that 50% of patients will test negative and will not need further intervention.
3. Reassure patients who are carrying a low risk.
4. Provide ongoing support for high-risk patients, ensuring that screening interventions are offered.

Case study

Mrs Poole, age 54, presented to her GP with a concern about her risk of breast cancer. Her mother had developed breast cancer when she was 82 and had died from a stroke 1 year later. Mrs Poole's sister, aged 60, had also recently been diagnosed with breast cancer. The GP took a full family history, consulted referral guidelines produced by the local department of clinical genetics and discussed these with Mrs Poole.

The GP explained to Mrs Poole that, although this family history might slightly increase her risk of breast cancer, no special interventions were indicated and she did not need to be referred. As breast cancer is a common disease, it was possible for two members of the same family to develop the disease without a strong hereditary element.

The GP reminded Mrs Poole to continue to attend for regular mammography and stressed she should report any further cancers developing in members of her family because this might affect the advice that the GP had given. Mrs Poole said that she was very relieved by the doctor's advice.

---

to evaluate whether the family history could fit with a single gene disorder–dominant, recessive or X-linked. Alternatively, for diseases in which only a small percentage of cases are caused by a mutant gene, it is necessary to ask whether it fulfils the criteria for referral for further assessment; breast and bowel cancer are examples here (Box 1 and Case study).

Screening

Screening for genetic problems in primary care is most frequently undertaken as pre-conception advice or in the antenatal booking clinic. The GP or midwife should be aware of high-risk cases, for example where a previous pregnancy has been affected by a single gene disorder or where a parent carries a balanced chromosome translocation. These women should be referred to secondary care for counselling before they become pregnant or in the early stages of pregnancy.

Most low-risk women will also be offered screening tests for genetic conditions – usually a combination of the nuchal translucency scan or the triple test for Down syndrome and an anomaly ultrasound scan. A woman should be carefully counselled before she undertakes these tests; she should be clear that a positive test could lead to further tests including an amniocentesis, with its risk of inducing miscarriage, or to the offer of a

termination. In the case of the triple test, she should be aware that the test is not diagnostic, women with a very low risk on the test still having a small chance of carrying a child with Down syndrome. A woman opposed to termination may prefer to avoid these tests.

The Guthrie test for the autosomal recessive condition phenylketonuria is routinely undertaken on newborn babies. The test looks for a biochemical marker for the condition so is usually not considered to be a genetic test.

Trials of population screening for carriers of autosomal recessive conditions have been undertaken in general practice. Conditions screened for include cystic fibrosis and thalassaemia in relevant ethnic populations. These trials have shown that screening is feasible in primary care and acceptable to patients, but the uptake is variable. There are currently no national screening programmes for these diseases but some are planned.

Table 2 Referral guidelines for potentially inherited cancers

A GP should consider the referral of a patient for further assessment any patient with one of the following family histories or worse:

Breast/ovarian cancer

- 3 first or second degree relatives with breast or ovarian cancer diagnosed at any age on the same side of the family
- 2 first or second degree relatives with breast cancer diagnosed under 60 or ovarian cancer at any age, on the same side of the family
- 1 first degree female relative with breast cancer diagnosed under 40
- A1 first degree male relative with breast cancer diagnosed at any age
- A first degree relative with bilateral breast cancer

Colorectal cancer

- 3 first or second degree relatives (one must be first degree) affected at any age on the same side of the family
- 2 first or second degree relatives (one must be first degree) both diagnosed under 60
- One first degree relative diagnosed under 45

Genetics in primary care

- Primary care will have an increasing role to play in the diagnosis and management of genetic conditions.

- There are two special considerations when making a genetic diagnosis: that

most genetic mutations are currently unalterable and that the diagnosis has implications for the relatives as well as the patient.

- The family history (pedigree) is the most important tool for

diagnosing a genetic disease.

- A GP's main role in clinical genetics currently lies in the areas of inherited cancers and antenatal screening.

Research in primary care

Research has been described as the 'systematic investigation and study of materials, sources, etc in order to establish facts and reach conclusions', 'an endeavour to discover facts by scientific study' and 'organised curiosity'. Research in primary care is relatively under-developed compared will hospital-based and laboratory research. There is huge potential here that has only recently begun to be realised, partly as a result of the belated recognition of its importance (Table 1). Three categories of primary care research have been described (Table 2).

History

Although primary care research is under-developed, there has been a long tradition of research carried out by GPs, usually conducted within their own practices. Edward Jenner, who developed vaccination, was a GP in Somerset, and important discoveries relating to yellow fever and typhoid were made by the GPs Finlay and Budd in the 19th century. John Snow and Robert Koch contributed to major advances in the areas of public health and infectious diseases. In the 20th century, pioneering work in cardiology and the epidemiology of infectious hepatitis was conducted by James McKenzie and William Pickles respectively. More recently, John Fry, Keith Hodgkin, Geoffrey Marsh, David Morrell and Julian Tudor-Hart have made significant contributions.

Within the past 20–30 years, research by individual GPs has been complemented by large multi-centre clinical trials, such as the oral contraceptive study from the Royal College of General Practitioners (RCGP), and collaborative, multi-disciplinary projects involving researchers from other backgrounds such as nursing, education, psychology, anthropology and sociology. Primary care research now involves biomedical science, social sciences, the humanities and organisational sciences, and embraces many methodologies, covering a spectrum ranging from qualitative to quantitative approaches.

Scope of primary care research

Because of its diversity and generalist orientation, primary care offers a huge range of options for research:

- clinical medicine
- the organisation and delivery of care
- social and behavioural issues, including the implementation of evidence in practice.

The quantitative approach lends itself to epidemiological research and clinical trials, and is used predominantly in biomedical research; it is strongly identified with the biomedical and reductionist models of health care (see p. 6). Issues of selection, randomisation, sample size and power are critical here (Table 3). The qualitative approach is more involved with the social world and social, cultural and psychological phenomena, and is identified with the biopsychosocial and holistic models of health care (see Section 1.3); it requires a different range of methods (Table 4).

The qualitative and quantitative approaches complement one another, each having its own strengths and weaknesses. Quantitative research poses hypotheses and endeavours to answer specific questions by collecting objective data that are subject to statistical analysis. It is strongly culture bound and therefore reflects the norms and values of Western society. Qualitative research is, in contrast, concerned with context, meaning, beliefs, behaviour and the social and cultural aspects of life, but it can be subject to observer error and disagreement. Primary care provides an ideal setting in which to combine the two approaches.

Funding and support

Compared with hospital and laboratory-based disciplines, primary care receives significantly fewer resources. Only 7% of the NHS research and development budget, and less than 5% of Medical Research Council (MRC) project funding, is spent on primary care research. The main sources of funding and support for research are:

1. the NHS R&D programme
2. research councils, especially the MRC

Table 1 **Reasons for supporting R&D in primary care**

- Decisions made in primary care need to be based on research evidence
- Primary care is central to the NHS and to individual patient care
- The evidence base for primary care needs to be strengthened
- Much of the evidence required for primary care can only be obtained by research in primary care involving primary care practitioners and their patients
- The capacity of primary care to undertake the R&D necessary to provide a firm evidence base is at present limited
- The appropriate involvement of primary care staff in R&D is likely to increase the quality of clinical care in the NHS
- Evidence-based health care must cross professional boundaries
- R&D in primary care is important to public health
- R&D is important to empower patients to make informed choices

Source: National Working Group on Research and Development in Primary Care (1997)

Table 2 **Categories of primary care research**

- Research initiated in primary care in which at least one principal investigator is a primary care professional – research *by* primary care practitioners
- Research initiated by others but in which patient recruitment and data collection are mainly carried out in primary care – research *through* primary care
- Research initiated and carried out by others but relating specifically to the activities of primary health-care professionals – research *on* primary care

Source: National Working Group on Research and Development in Primary Care (1997)

Table 3 **Some examples of quantitative research methods**

- Meta-analyses
- Randomised controlled trials
- Cohort studies
- Case-control studies
- Cross-sectional studies
- Morbidity surveys

Table 4 **Some examples of qualitative research methods**

- Participant observation
- Non-participant observation
- Unstructured interviews
- Semi-structured interviews
- Focused interviews
- Ethnology
- Ethnograpy
- Pathography
- Ethnomethodology
- Content analysis (some forms of)

Source: Bradley (1998)

3. medical charities and trusts, for example the British Heart Foundation, the Wellcome Trust, the British Diabetic Association and the Nuffield Provincial Hospitals Trust
4. academic departments of general practice and primary health care
5. the RCGP
6. private foundations, industry and pharmaceutical companies.

The NHS R&D programme, established in 1991, aims to spend 1.5% of the total NHS budget on research and to 'create a knowledge-based health service in which clinical, managerial and policy decisions are based on sound information about research findings and scientific developments' (Department of Health 1993).

There is a central programme of commissioned research and within nationally commissioned R&D programmes, the breakdown of expenditure by primary care discipline is:

■ general practice 76%
■ nursing 7%
■ midwifery 5%
■ pharmacy 5%
■ health visiting 3%
■ dentistry 3%
■ optometry <1%
■ professions allied to medicine <1%.

As well as funding specific research projects, the NHS R&D programme provides support for research training and infrastructure, including research networks and research practices (see below).

The MRC has recently developed a new funding structure and has encouraged primary care researchers to apply for group development and programme support. It also provides junior and senior research training posts and supports a network of over 900 practices that contribute to large-scale clinical trials.

A small amount of funding is provided by medical charities and trusts, but most of their resources support hospital and laboratory-based research.

The RCGP provides support in the form of:

■ research training fellowships
■ research practices
■ RCGP research units – the Birmingham unit, for example, conducts the National Morbidity Survey (a 10-yearly study of patients'

consulting behaviour) and the Aberdeen unit focuses on contraception and cardiovascular disease

■ advice and publications, including the *British Journal of General Practice*
■ small grants through its Scientific Foundation Board (SFB).

All medical schools now have departments of general practice or primary health care, and there are also postgraduate departments and primary care/general practice/health services research units associated with many universities and health authorities. These various institutions offer opportunities for higher research degrees (MD, PhD, MPhil) and advice, training and support for primary care researchers.

In order for primary care research to develop its full potential, there needs to be a considerable increase in the number and skills of researchers. Strong recommendations for additional training and infrastructural support have been made in two recent reports, from the MRC (1997) and the National Working Group on R&D in Primary Care (1997), and the government has promised to double the spending on primary care R&D over the next 5 years.

Research practices and networks

The RCGP, the NHS R&D programme and the Scottish Office now support what are known as 'research general practices'. The funding ranges from £4500 to £20 000 per annum for 2–3 years and is not intended to fund research projects but to buy protected time, training and equipment for the practice. Research general practices have been established in order to develop research capacity in primary health care and to facilitate the establishment of a research culture in the community. They are based on the premise that 'those working within

general practice will produce high quality research evidence from within primary care that will improve patient care' (Smith 1997).

There are currently almost 50 primary care research networks throughout the country, many of which incorporate research practices. They vary in size (from 10 individuals to over 900 practices) and sophistication, and there is now a National Federation of Primary Care Research Networks to bring together this considerable experience and expertise. The strategic purpose of networks is:

■ to encourage and facilitate collaborative R&D
■ to support primary care practitioners in conducting their own R&D.

Implementation

Although new research evidence is constantly being generated, there is often a considerable delay in this evidence being implemented in clinical practice. There are many reasons for this, including a lack of appropriate information at the point of decision-making, and social, organisational and institutional barriers to change (Haines and Donald 1998).

There is no simple solution to this problem, and a number of approaches are needed (Haines and Donald 1998), including:

■ employing evidence-based guidelines
■ using computerised decision support systems
■ developing educational programmes
■ communicating research findings to patients
■ developing strategies for organisational change
■ influencing opinion leaders.

Such an integrated approach will require the development of closer links between research, continuing education, audit and clinical practice.

Research in primary care

■ Research is needed to underpin the evolution of primary care, but is currently underdeveloped compared with hospital based and laboratory research.
■ Primary care embraces a

wide range of disciplines and offers a diverse and broad setting for research, suitable for both qualitative and quantitative approaches.
■ General practice accounts for over 75% of NHS primary

care R&D expenditure.
■ Research general practices and primary care research networks are key components in developing research capacity in primary care.

Appendix 1 **Examples of some common medicines**

Therapeutic group	Main use	Example(s) of drugs in this group: generic (proprietary) names	Examples of possible adverse effects
H_2-receptor antagonists	Reduce stomach acid production. Used to treat gastric and duodenal ulcers	Cimetidene (Tagamet), ranitidine (Zantac)	Not common, but may cause, for example, diarrhoea, headache and tiredness. Cimetidine can interfere with the effect of other medicines
Corticosteroids ('steroids')	Suppress any kind of inflammation. Used, for example, as tablets, inhalers, creams for rheumatoid arthritis, in asthma and for skin diseases	Prednisolone is most common tablet form. Inhalers such as beclometasone (Becotide). Creams such as betamethasone (Betnovate)	Taking steroid tablets (especially for a long period) can cause stomach ulcers, weight gain and high blood pressure, among many other effects that include the stunting of growth in children
Cardiac glycosides	Increase the force of heart muscle contraction and thus assist patients with heart failure	Digoxin (Lanoxin), a synthetic form of extract of foxglove leaves	Can cause stomach upset followed by serious heart irregularities if too much accumulates in the body
Diuretics	Counteract water retention. Used in heart failure and high blood pressure	Bendrofluazide, furosemide (frusemide) (Lasix)	Can cause patients to develop diabetes and gout
Beta-adrenoceptor blockers ('beta-blockers')	Block some of the stimulant effects of the body's adrenaline system. Used for high blood pressure and heart disease	Propranolol (Inderal), atenolol (Tenormin)	Can cause the hands and feet to be very cold because of decreased bood circulation and can cause asthma in those predisposed to it
Nitrates	Increase the blood supply to the heart muscle. Used for chest pain caused by angina	Glyceryl trinitrate, as tablets, spray or skin patches	May cause headache and temporary faintness
Lipid-regulating drugs	Lower blood cholesterol	Statins are the most frequently used type, e.g. simvastatin (Zocor)	Statins can cause stomach upset and headache. They very rarely cause inflammation of the muscles, leading to pain and weakness.
Beta$_2$-adrenoceptor stimulants	Dilate the airways. Mainly used for quick relief in asthma	Salbutamol (Ventolin)	If used excessively, salbutamol can cause acute anxiety-like symptoms
Anxiolytics and sedatives	Mainly benzodiazepines (which are also commonly abused by addicts)	Diazepam (Valium), temazepam	The main dangers are dependence and abuse of these drugs
Antidepressants	Two main groups of drug are used in general practice to treat depression	Tricyclics – e.g. amitryptiline. SSRIs – e.g. fluoxetine (Prozac)	Tricyclics are dangerous in overdose (particularly in children) and may rarely have serious effects on the heart in patients with existing heart disease. SSRIs are generally thought to be safer but may occasionally cause bleeding (e.g. in the stomach)
Analgesics	These are the drugs used to treat pain, although NSAIDs are also used	The main groups are non-opioids, mainly aspirin and paracetamol, and opioids, e.g. codeine and morphine	Aspirin can cause stomach ulcers and bleeding from the gut, and paracetamol causes severe liver damage in overdose. Opioids are varyingly addictive depending on their potency (codeine being the weakest)
NSAIDs	Several different kinds of chemical group (of which aspirin is the original) counteract inflammation but are not steroids. They are used mainly in rheumatic conditions	Ibuprofen (Brufen), diclofenac (Voltarol)	NSAIDs can aggravate asthma and heart failure, but the most common adverse effect is irritation of the stomach, leading to ulcers or bleeding
Antibiotics	Treat infections	Penicillins, erythromycin and tetracyclines	Most antibiotics can cause stomach upsets and encourage thrush (a simple yeast infection) to develop, especially in the vagina in women
Female sex hormones	Used in OCPs and HRT	OCPs: Logynon, Femulen. HRT: Prempak-C	These are generally thought to be relatively safe. OCP use is more risky in older women who smoke

SSRI, selective serotonin re-uptake inhibitor; NSAID, non-steroidal anti-inflammatory drugs; OCP, oral contraceptive pills; HRT, hormone replacement therapy.

Appendix 2 **An example of a morning surgery**

It is difficult to give a generalisable example of a typical 'surgery' or session of GP consultations because there are so many factors affecting the 'case-mix' or kinds of patients and problems that will be dealt with. For example, the geographical location will affect what diseases are commonest in that area. What is common in an underdeveloped tropical country will be quite different from what is common in a temperate industrialised country like the UK. But even within a country there are big geographical variations, mainly because of differences in the overall wealth of different areas, and the mix between rich and relatively poor people. Different illnesses also predominate at different times of the year. In the UK, for example, influenza and other respiratory infections tend to predominate over the winter months. Even within a single general practice, however, there can still be big variations in the case-mix of surgeries. Many female patients want to see a female doctor about intimate problems, and the same may apply to males. Doctors tend to "get old with their patients" i.e. older doctors tend to see older patients and vice versa. The surgeries of the well established, more experienced doctors are taken up more with chronic illness and review appointments whilst less established doctors, trainees and locums, who have not yet built up their own clientele, will tend to be more available to see patients who want to see any doctor quickly, usually because they have an acute illness. Bearing all this in mind, one of us (RJT) gives the following illustration of a fairly typical surgery for him – a well established older doctor with an interest in child health. Each appointment is scheduled for 10 minutes and it is a Wednesday morning in November ….

We have not been able to avoid using some technical terms here which are not all covered in the book itself. Where you want to find out more the best plan will be to ask your tutor. It isn't necessary to know what some of these terms mean because we are only trying to give an illustration of 'case-mix'.

Mr & Mrs A. These are a couple well into their 70s who are quite fit for their age but have a number of ongoing health problems. They relate to me almost as personal friends because we have known each other for many years and they attend regularly. They are mainly here to check on results of tests and reports from hospital appointments. Mrs A is in the throes of having investigation of her liver and gall bladder. Mr A had a prostatectomy a few years ago and is now having some urinary problems again.

Mrs B (43 years old). She had severe endometriosis for which she had some surgical treatment (endometriosis is a troublesome gynaecological condition causing pain and menstrual problems) and has a previous history of urinary infections. Both cause similar symptoms at times so she has come mainly to clarify whether she has a urinary infection or not and to get the treatment she needs.

Mr C (42 years old). He had a lesion on his nose, which my partner very promptly diagnosed as a basal cell carcinoma (see p. 57). He is now worried about some other spots of various kinds on his body (not surprising really when you have had this kind of fright) but I examine them all carefully and am able to reassure him that they are all quite harmless. I then also outline to him what to look out for himself in any new skin blemish.

Child D (2.5 years old). He was sick during the night, woke up crying and felt very hot to touch. I examine him very gently but thoroughly because this could be any kind of infection. He has no neck stiffness or rashes, which helps to exclude meningitis along with the fact that he does have a very inflamed Rt eardrum (acute otitis media – see p. 39), which is sufficient to account for his symptoms.

Miss E (26 years old). She asks for a repeat prescription for her contraceptive pill, but she could have got that without seeing me. This suggests that there might be some other reason why she is here. It turns out that she is not sleeping well and is feeling down and even depressed at times, but can't understand why, because nothing special has happened. I generally encourage her to talk about herself and try to establish how severe this depression is and what it might be due to (including her oral contraceptive). I will probably have to see her again a few times before we resolve what treatment (if any) is needed.

Mr F (32 years old). He was playing amateur football at the weekend when he injured his Lt knee. The knee is still swollen and painful, but is getting better. It looks like he may have injured a 'cartilage' in his knee – a common footballer's injury.

Mr G (45 years old). He is an insulin-dependent diabetic. He wants treatment for a persistent cough. He seems to have a 'chest infection' for which I prescribe treatment. This will need to be followed up but I also note that he has not been attending regularly for diabetic checkups and has not been to the specialist diabetic clinic for a considerable time. I order some tests and discuss with him at length the importance of these things.

Miss H (24 years old). She has had a cough and sore throat for only a few days. Her symptoms aren't severe but because she is a nurse in an intensive care unit she has been told to go off work and see a doctor so that she does not pass infections on to patients.

Mr I (38 years old). He is scruffily dressed and unkempt and I know that he should be on long-term treatment for schizophrenia (see p. 72). He had been doing well and actually holding down a job as a packer in a food factory. It isn't very clear what he wants because his speech and general thought processes are difficult to follow. It seems he hasn't been taking his medication. This all needs to be sorted out quite urgently and takes up more time than has been allocated.

Child J (12 years old). A boy has been brought in direct to our treatment (emergency) room with severe breathlessness. He is one of our known quite severe asthmatics. Our nurse has already started him on emergency treatment but I need to break my surgery to go and help her stabilise this patient. Fortunately he is very soon dramatically better.

Mrs K (49 years old). She is feeling very down and depressed, something she has had a lot of trouble with before over the years. She has had antidepressant treatment a number of times. She also has profuse sweating attacks and other menopausal symptoms. There are a number of possible approaches to treatment here and again it will probably take several consultations to come to a conclusion about what is best for this individual.

This whole session has taken just under 2 hours and there is still a bit of paperwork to do …

Appendix 3 **Common sports injuries**

Site	Examples of injury
Eye	Direct injury e.g. from squash and golf balls, may cause blindness
Ear	Heavy blows to the ear cause bruising and 'cauliflower ear'
Nose	Is the most commonly broken bone in the face
Intracranial injury	Boxers particularly suffer from chronic brain injury – the 'punch drunk' syndrome
The neck	Acute torticollis – spasm of the neck muscles due to injury
	More seriously – permanent paralysis can result from injury to the spinal cord in the neck e.g. from diving, rugby, hang gliding etc.
Shoulder and upper arm	Dislocations and fractures. 'Overuse' syndromes – inflammation of tendons and other soft tissue
Lumbar spine	Lumbar disc injuries. Long term, possibly increased risk of osteoarthritis
Elbow and forearm	'Tennis elbow' and 'Golfer's elbow', fractures especially of the radius, dislocation of elbow
Wrist and hand	Tenosynovitis from overuse, fractures especially of the wrist
Pelvis and thigh	Muscle strains, especially of adductor muscles in inner thigh
Knees	Very susceptible to injury of tendons, cartilages and joint itself
Legs	Fractures of leg bones (skiing etc); rupture of tendons e.g. Achilles tendon
Feet	Plantar fasciitis; stress fractures of small bones of foot

Appendix 4 **Some of the essential features of a UK National Health Service (NHS) prescription**

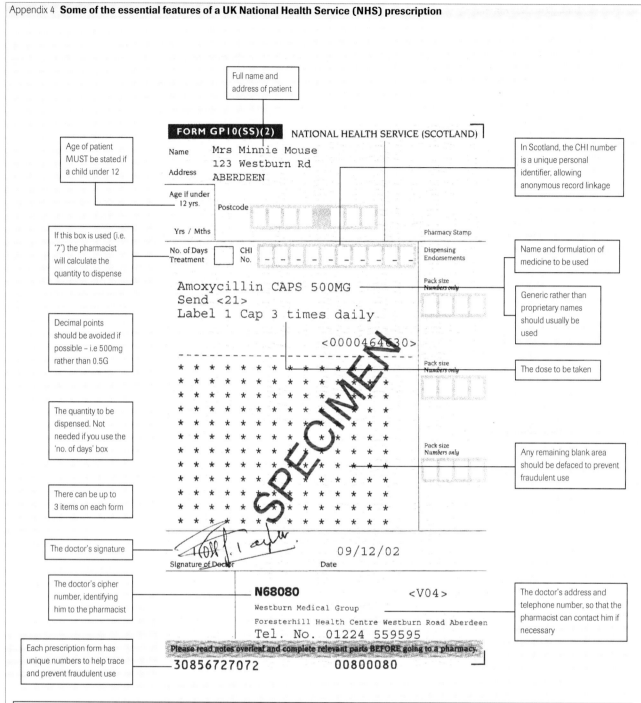

Full name and address of patient

Age of patient MUST be stated if a child under 12

In Scotland, the CHI number is a unique personal identifier, allowing anonymous record linkage

If this box is used (i.e. '7') the pharmacist will calculate the quantity to dispense

Name and formulation of medicine to be used

Decimal points should be avoided if possible – i.e 500mg rather than 0.5G

Generic rather than proprietary names should usually be used

The dose to be taken

The quantity to be dispensed. Not needed if you use the 'no. of days' box

Any remaining blank area should be defaced to prevent fraudulent use

There can be up to 3 items on each form

The doctor's signature

The doctor's cipher number, identifying him to the pharmacist

The doctor's address and telephone number, so that the pharmacist can contact him if necessary

Each prescription form has unique numbers to help trace and prevent fraudulent use

FORM GP10(SS)(2) NATIONAL HEALTH SERVICE (SCOTLAND)

Name   Mrs Minnie Mouse
Address 123 Westburn Rd
         ABERDEEN

Age if under 12 yrs.   Postcode

Yrs / Mths

No. of Days Treatment   CHI No.   Dispensing Endorsements

Pharmacy Stamp

Amoxycillin CAPS 500MG
Send <21>
Label 1 Cap 3 times daily

<0000464630>

Pack size Numbers only

SPECIMEN

Signature of Doctor   Date   09/12/02

N68080   <V04>

Westburn Medical Group
Foresterhill Health Centre Westburn Road Aberdeen
Tel. No. 01224 559595

Please read notes overleaf and complete relevant parts BEFORE going to a pharmacy.

30856727072   00800080

Notes:
1 This is a version of the Scottish NHS prescription form. The versions used in other countries (including within the UK) are slightly different NB: this is not an actual replica of a prescription form.
2 This is a form for use by a general (medical) practitioner, but nurses and pharmacists may issue certain kinds of NHS prescription on similar forms, especially marked for their use.

Appendix 5 **Meningitis and septicaemia symptom checklist**

Meningitis & Septicaemia can kill in hours – know the symptoms

Rash (develops anywhere on body)	Fever/ vomiting	Cold hands and feet	Rapid breathing	Stomach/joint/ muscle pain	Drowsiness/ impaired consciousness	Severe headache	Stiff neck	Dislike of bright lights

Septicaemia Symptoms

✓	✓	✓	✓	Sometimes with diarrhoea ✓	Not in all cases ✓			

Meningitis Symptoms

Not present in all cases ✓	✓				✓	✓	Unusual in young children ✓	Unusual in young children ✓

Babies may also suffer from:	**Tumbler test**
• tense or bulging soft spot on their head • blotchy skin, getting paler or turning blue • refusing to feed • irritable when picked up, with a high pitched or moaning cry • a stiff body with jerky movements, or else floppy and lifeless	If a glass tumbler is pressed firmly against a septicaemic rash, the rash will not fade. You will be able to see the rash through the glass. If this happens get medical help immediately.

Symptoms can occur in any order. Not everyone gets all these symptoms. Septicaemia can occur with or without meningitis.

Remember....trust your instincts. Someone who has meningitis or septicaemia needs medical help urgently.

This is an example of a card produced by the Meningitis Research Foundation, UK. Reproduced with permission.

Appendix 6 **Accidental injury in children**

Injury	Examples of preventive measures
Road accidents are the commonest cause of death in childhood	Reduce bicycle accidents – e.g. training, cycle helmets and good machines; bright reflective clothing; in car restraints and child seats; road safety training; safe road arrangements – crossings etc.
Falls	Stairgates, safe windows, prevent small children climbing onto high furniture etc.
Fires and scalds	Fireguards and cooker guard to prevent tipping of pots. Keep matches out of reach
Medicines and poisoning	Lock up medicines and poisons. Many look like sweets. Iron pills and antidepressants are especially dangerous. Many household chemicals are very poisonous
Playground injuries	Playgrounds should be made safe with well designed swings for different ages, soft landing areas, slides incorporated into grassy banks. Limbs or clothing can be caught in unsafe roundabouts
Unsafe environments	It is better to get rid of the hazards as far as possible i.e make houses, streets and schools safe environments for children rather than depend on them avoiding hazards (although that should also be taught). Railway tracks and waterways are particularly difficult to make entirely safe
Other hazards	Small objects e.g. tyres from model cars can be inhaled – inhaled peanuts are especially dangerous; plastic bags can suffocate. All should be kept well away from small children

Bibliography

Importance and relevance of primary health care

Fry J, Sandler G 1993 Common diseases, 5th edn. Klumer Academic, London

Ljubljana Charter on Reforming Health Care 1996 WHO, Geneva

McWhinney I R 1997 A textbook of family medicine, 2nd edn. Oxford University Press, Oxford

Royal College of General Practitioners Welsh Council and Welsh General Medical Services Committee 1994 Patient care and the general practitioner. A discussion document. Department of Postgraduate Studies, University of Wales College of Medicine, Cardiff

Starfield B 1992 Primary care: concept, evaluation and policy. Oxford University Press, Oxford

Tarimo E, Webster E G 1994 Primary health care concepts and challenges in a changing world. Alma Ata revisited. World Health Organization – Division of Strengthening of Health Services: 11

Vuori H 1986 Health for all, primary health care and general practitioners. Journal of the Royal College of General Practitioners 35: 398–402

World Health Organization 1971 The role of the primary physician in health services. Report of a conference, Noordwijk-ann-Zee, 1970. WHO, Copenhagen

World Health Organization 1978 Primary health care. WHO, Geneva

Overview and philosophy of generalist practice

Feinstein A 1983 An additional basic science for clinical medicine. The constraining fundamental paradigms. Annals of Internal Medicine 99: 393–397

Fraser R C (ed.) 1999 Clinical method: a general practice approach, 3rd edn. Butterworth–Heinemann, Oxford

Marinker M 1990 General practice and the new contract. In Bevan G, Marinker M (eds) Greening the White Paper. Social Market Foundation, London

McWhinney I R 1997 A textbook of family medicine, 2nd edn. Oxford University Press, Oxford

Office of Populations, Censuses and Surveys 1995 Morbidity statistics from general practice – 4th national study 1991/92. OPCS, London

Royal College of General Practitioners 1996 The nature of general medicine practice. Report from general practice no. 27. RCGP, London

Spence J 1960 The purpose and practice of medicine. Oxford University Press, Oxford

Models of health care

Engel G L 1980 The clinical application of the biopsychosocial model. American Journal of Psychiatry 137; 535–544

General Medical Council 2002 Tomorrow's doctors. Recommendations on undergraduate medical education. GMC, London

McWhinney I R 1989 An acquaintance with particulars … . Family Medicine, 21:296–298

Spence J 1960 The purpose and practice of medicine. Oxford University Press, Oxford

Stewart M, Brown J, Weston W et al 1995 Patient-centred medicine. Sage, California

Toon P 1994 What is good general practice? Occasional paper no. 65. Royal College of General Practitioners, London

Tuckett D, Boulton M, Olson C, Williams A 1985 Meetings between experts: an approach to sharing ideas in medical consultations. Tavistock, London

International Comparisons I and II

Bass M J, Buck C W, Turner L et al 1986 The physician's action and the outcome of illness in family practice. Journal of Family Practice 23: 43

Bridges–Webb C, Britt H, Miles D A, Neary S, Charles J, Traynor V 1992 Morbidity and treatment in general practice in Australia 1990–1991. Medical Journal of Australia 158:51–56

Fry J, Horder J P 1994 Primary health care in an international context. Nuffield Provisional Hospitals Trust, London

Kabayashi Y 1997 Development of primary care in Japan. Proceedings of International Symposium on suggestions for primary care physicians in Japan. Japanese Association of Primary Care, Tokyo

McAvoy B R, Davis P, Raymont A, Gribben B 1994 The Waikato medical care (WaiMedCa) survey 1991–1992. New Zealand Medical Journal 107(5):386–433

Organisation for Economic Co-operation and Development 2001 The OECD in 2001. OECD, Paris

Rakel R E 1997 Viewpoint of a family physician. Proceedings of international symposium on suggestions for primary care physicians in Japan. Japanese Association of Primary Care, Tokyo

Rosenblatt R A, Hart L G, Gamliel S, Goldstein B, McLenden B J 1995 Identifying primary care disciplines by analysing the diagnostic content of ambulatory care. Journal of the American Board of Family Practice 8:34–45

Royal College of General Practitioners 1992

The European study of referrals from primary to secondary care. Occasional paper no. 56. Royal College of General Practitioners, London

Starfield B 1992 Primary care: concept, evaluation and policy. Oxford University Press, Oxford

Starfield B 1994 Is primary care essential? Lancet, 344:1129–1133

Wilkin D, Hallam L, Leavey R, Metcalfe D 1987 Anatomy of urban general practice. Tavistock, London

World Health Organization 2001 The world health report 2000 – Health systems: improving performance. World Health Organization, Geneva

Resources and needs: UK perspective I and II

Baker M 1998 Making sense of the new NHS White Paper. Radcliffe Medical Press, Oxford

Berwick D M 1998 The NHS: feeling well and thriving at 75. BMJ, 317:57–61

Department of Health 1998 Our Healthier Nation: a contract for health. Department of Health, London

Department of Health (DOH) 2000 Health and personal social services statistics England. Government Statistical Service, London

Department of Health/Royal College of General Practitioners 2002 Implementing a scheme for General Practitioners with Special Interests. DOH/RCGP, London

Harrison J, van Zwanenberg T 1998 GP tomorrow. Radcliffe Medical Press, Oxford

Lewis R, Gillam S 2002 A fresh new contract for general practitioners. BMJ, 324:1048–1049

Office of Health Economics 2000 Twelfth compendium of health statistics. Office of Health Economics, London

Royal College of General Practitioners 1992 Conference on Primary Health Care, September 1991. In Royal College of General Practitioner, Members' Reference Book 1992. Sabrecrown Publishing, London

Royal College of General Practitioners 1996 The nature of general medical practice. Report from general practice no. 27. Royal College of General Practitioners, London

Royal College of General Practitioners 1999 Profile of UK practices. Information sheet no. 2. Royal College of General Practitioners, London

Royal College of General Practitioners 2000 Profile of UK general practitioners. Information sheet no. 1. Royal College of General Practitioners, London

Royal College of General Practitioners 2001 General practitioners workload. Information sheet no. 3. Royal College of General Practitioners, London

Scally G, Donaldson L J 1998 Clinical governance and the drive for quality improvement in the new NHS in England. British Medical Journal 317:61–65

Secretary of State for Health 1996 Primary care: the future. Department of Health, London

Secretary of State for Health 2001 The NHS Plan. A plan for investment. A plan for reform. Department of Health, London

Professional standards

British Medical Association 1993 Medical ethics today. British Medical Journal Publishing Group, London

Department of Health 2000 The NHS plan. HMSO, London

General Medical Council 1995 Duties of a doctor. Guidance from the General Medical Council. General Medical Council, London

Royal College of General Practitioners 1999 Clinical governance: practical advice for primary care in England and Wales. Royal College of General Practitioners, London

Evidence-based medicine

Barton S (ed) Clinical evidence. British Medical Journal Publishing Group, London

Barton S 2000 Which clinical studies provide the best evidence? British Medical Journal 321: 255–256

Barton S 2001 Using clinical evidence? British Medical Journal 322: 503–504

Greenhalgh T 1997 How to read a paper: the basics of evidence based medicine. British Medical Journal Publications

McColl A, Smith H, White P, Field J 1998 General practitioners' perceptions of the route to evidence based medicine: a questionnaire survey. British Medical Journal 316: 361–365

Sackett D L, Straus S, Richardson S, Rosenberg W, Haynes R B 2000 Evidence-based medicine: how to practice and teach EBM (2nd edn) Churchill Livingstone, London

Inequalities in health

Acheson D (Chairman) 1998 Report of the independent inquiry into inequalities in health. Stationery Office, London

Benzeval M, Judge K, Whitehead M 1977 Tackling inequalities in health. An agenda for action. King's Fund, London

Johnson Z, Howell F, Molloy B 1993 Community mothers' programme: Randomised controlled trial of professional intervention in parenting. British Medical Journal 306:1449–1452

Office of Population Censuses and Surveys 1993 General household survey. HMSO, London

Registrar General 1991 Registrar General's decennial supplements and mortality tables. HMSO, London

Tudor Hart J 1971 The inverse care law. Lancet (i): 405–412

World Health Organization 1998 The solid facts. World Health Organization, www.who.dk

Family medicine

Benzeval M, Judge K, Whitehead M (eds) 1995 Tackling inequalities in health: an agenda for action. King's Fund, London

Bowlby J 1969 Attachment and loss, vol. 1. Hogarth Press, London

Duvall E M 1977 Family development, 5th edn. JB Lippincott, Philadelphia

Falloon I R H, Laporta M, Fadden G, Graham-Hole V 1993 Managing stress in families. Routledge, London

Henderson A S 1988 An introduction to social psychiatry. Oxford University Press, Oxford

Hull D, Johnston D I 1993 Essential paediatrics. Churchill Livingstone, Edinburgh

Huygen F J A 1990 Family medicine: the medical life history of families. Royal College of General Practitioners, London

McWhinney I R 1981 An introduction to family medicine. Oxford University Press, Oxford

Rakel R E 1977 Principles of family medicine. W B Saunders, Philadelphia

Changes in society

Dickson N, Paul C, Herbison P, Silva P 1998 First sexual intercourse: age, coercion, and later regrets reported by a birth cohort. British Medical Journal 316: 29–33

Hall A H with Webb J (eds) 2000 Twentieth century British social trends. Palgrave, London

Johnson A M, Wadsworth J, Wellings K, Field J 1994 Sexual attitudes and lifestyles. Blackwell Science, London

Todd J, Currie C, Smith R 1999 Health behaviours of Scottish schoolchildren. Technical report 2: Sexual health in the 1990s. Research Unit in Health and Behavioural Change, University of Edinburgh, Edinburgh

Wight D, Henderson M, Raab G et al 2000 Extent of regretted sexual intercourse among young teenagers in Scotland: a cross sectional survey. British Medical Journal 320: 1243–1244

Risks and health

Dhalgren G, Whitehead M 1991 Policies and strategies to promote social equity in health. Institute for Futures Studies, Stockholm

Laupacis A, Sackett D L, Roberts R S 1988 New England Journal of Medicine 318: 1728–1733

General principles

Holland W, Dettels R, George Knox G (eds) 1991 Oxford textbook of public health, vol. 3. Oxford Medical Publications, Oxford

Practical issues

Family Heart Study Group. 1994 Randomised controlled trial evaluating cardiovascular screening and intervention in general practice: principal results of the British Family Heart Study. British Medical Journal 308:313–320

Prochaska J O, DiClemente C C 1992 Stages of change in the modification of problem behaviours. Prog Behav Motif 28:183–218

Skrabanek P, McCormick J S 1998 Follies and fallacies in medicine, 3rd edn. Whithorn Tarragan Press

Stott N C H S, Davis R H 1979 The exceptional potential in each primary care consultation. Journal of the Royal College of General Practitioners 29:201–205

Children

Erikson E H 1968 Identify, use and crisis. Norton, New York

Stafford N D, Youngs R 1999 ENT Colour guide, 2nd edn. Churchill Livingstone, Edinburgh

Adults

Jones K, Moon G 1992 Health, disease and society. Routledge, London

Maslow A H 1954 Motivation and personality Harper & Row, New York

Panzer R J et al (eds) 1991 Diagnostic strategies for common medical problems. American College of Physicians, Philadelphia

Scottish Health Statistics 1991

The elderly

Forbes A 1996 Caring for old people: loneliness. British Medical Journal 313: 352–354

Hodkinson H M 1972 Evaluation of a mental test score for assessment of mental impairment in the elderly. British Medical Journal 1: 233–238

McMurdo M E T 2000 A healthy old age: realistic or futile goal? British Medical Journal 321: 1149–1151

Mann A 1996 Epidemiology. In Jacoby R, Oppenheimer C (eds), Psychiatry in the elderly. Oxford University Press, Oxford

Marlowe H 1994 Health trends in the last 75 years. Health Trends 26: 98–105

Mulley G P 1997 Myths of ageing. Lancet 350: 1160–1161

Office of National Statistics (ONS) 1996 Key date (1996 edition) HMSO, London

Men and women's health

Austoker J, Mansel R, Baum M, Sainsbury R, Hobbs R 1999 Guidelines for referral of patients with breast problems. NHS Breast Screening Porgramme, Sheffield

Guillebaud J 1999 Contraception your questions answered 3E. Churchill Livingstone, Edinburgh

McCormick A, Fleming D, Charlton J 1995 Morbidity statistics from General Practice. Fourth National Study 1991–1992. OPCS. HMSO, London

McPherson A 1993 Women's problems in general practice, 3rd edn. Oxford University Press, Oxford

Power D A, Brown R S, Brock C S, Payne H A, Majeed A, Babb P 2001 Trends in testicular carcinoma in England and Wales 1971–1999. British Journal of Urology 87(4):361–365

Preston-Whyte M E, Fraser R C, Beckett J L 1983 Effect of a principal's gender on consultation patterns. Journal of the Royal College of General Practitioners 255: 654–658

Prochaska J O, DiClemente C C 1992 Stages of change in the modification of problem behaviours. Prog Behav Modif. 28:183–218

Tannahill A 1985 What is health promotion? Health Education Journal 44: 167–168

Acute respiratory tract infections

Ellis M (ed.) 1998 Infectious diseases of the respiratory tract. Cambridge University Press, Cambridge

Infections and infestations of the skin

Gawkrodger D 2002 Dermatology. An illustrated colour text, 3rd edn. Churchill Livingstone, Edinburgh

White G 1997 Levene's colour atlas of dermatology 2E. Mosby, London

Wilkinson J D, Shaw S 1998 Dermatology Colour guide, 2E. Churchill Livingstone, Edinburgh

Chronic skin disease

Gawkrodger D J 2002 Dermatology 3E. Churchill Livingstone, Edinburgh

Marks R 1996 Practical problems in dermatology, 2nd edn. Martin Dunitz, London

Souhami R L, Moxham J (eds) 1997 Textbook of medicine, 3rd edn. Churchill Livingstone, Edinburgh

Obstructive airways disease

Panzer R J, Black E R, Griner P F (eds) 1991 Diagnostic strategies for common medical problems. American College of Physicians, Philadelphia

Souhami R L, Moxham J (eds) 2003 Textbook of medicine 4th edn. Churchill Livingstone, Edinburgh

Swash M (ed.) 1995 Hutchison's clinical methods. WB Saunders, London

Diabetes mellitus

DAWN study. www.dawnstudy.com

Forbes C D, Jackson W F 1991 Colour atlas and text of clinical medicine Mosby, London

Kinmonth A L, Griffen S, Wareham N J 1999 The implications of the United Kingdom Prospective Diabetes Study for general practice care of type 2 diabetes. British Journal of General Practice 49(446): 692–693

Office of Population Censuses and Surveys 1993

Pitts M, Phillips K (eds) 1998 The psychology of health. An introduction. Routledge, London

The Diabetes Control and Complications Research Group 1993 The effect of intensive treatment of diabetes on the development and progression of long-term complications in insulin-dependent diabetes mellitus. NEJM 329: 977–986

The Poole Diabetes Study 1999 The incidence prevalence and outcome of type 2 diabetes in a defined population. South West Research and Development Directorate,

UK Prospective Diabetes Study Group 1998 Intensive blood glucose control with sulphonylureas or insulin compared with conventional treatment and risk of complications in patients with type 2 diabetes. Lancet 352: 837–853

Hypertension

Boon N A, Fox K A A, Bloomfield P 2003 Diseases of the cardiovascular system. In: Haslett C, Chilvers E R, Hunter J A A, Boon N A (eds). Davidson's principles and practice of medicine, 19th edn. Churchill Livingstone, Edinburgh

Fry J, Sandler G 1993 Common diseases. Their nature, presentation and care, 5th edn. Kluwer Academic, London

Guidelines Subcommittee of the WHO-ISH 1999 WHO-ISH guidelines for the management of hypertension. Journal of Hypertension 17:151–183

National Blood Pressure Advisory Committee 1999 Guide to management of hypertension for doctors. National Heart Foundation of Australia, Canberra

Walker J M, Tan L B 2002 Cardiovascular disease. In: Souhami R L, Moxham J (eds) Textbook of medicine, 4th edn. Churchill Livingstone, Edinburgh

Common mental health problems

4th National Morbidity Study 1991–1992

Casey P R 1997 A guide to psychiatry in primary care, 2nd edn. Wrightson Biomedical, Petersfield, UK

Geddes J, Freemantle N, Harrison P, Bebbington 2000 Atypical antipsychotics and the treatment of schizophrenia: systematic overview and

meta regression analysis. BMJ 321:1371–1376

Gelder M, Gath D, Mayou R, Cowen P (eds) 1996 Oxford textbook of psychiatry, 3rd edn. Oxford University Press, Oxford

Guidelines Subcommittee of the WHO-ISH 1999 WHO-ISH guidelines for the managment of hypertension. Journal of Hypertension 17:151–183

Knesper D J, Riba M B, Schwenk T L (eds) 1997 Primary care psychiatry. W B Saunders, Philadelphia

Rees L, Lipsedge M, Bell C (eds) 1997 Textbook of psychiatry. Arnold, London

Sandifer M G 1972 Psychiatric diagnosis: cross-national research findings. Proceedings of the Royal Society of Medicine 65(5): 497–500

Wright A 1999 Through a glass darkly – understanding depression. British Journal of General Practice 49: 91–92

Heart disease

Boon N A, Fox K A A, Bloomfield P 2003 Diseases of cardiovascular system. In Haslett C, Chilvers E R, Hunter J A A, Boon N A (eds) 2003 Davidson's principles and practice of medicine, 19th edn. Churchill Livingstone, Edinburgh

Fry J, Sandler G. 1993 Common diseases. Their nature, presentation and care, 5th edn. Kluwer Academic, London

North of England Stable Angina Guideline Development Group 1996 North of England evidence based guideline development project: summary version of evidence based guideline for the primary care management of stable angina. British Medical Journal 312: 827–832

Walker J M, Tan L B 2002 Cardiovascular disease. In Souhami R L, Moxham J (eds) Textbook of medicine, 4th edn. Churchill Livingstone, Edinburgh

Chronic musculoskeletal disorders

Buschbacher R M (ed) 1994 Musculoskeletal disorders. A practical guide for diagnosis and rehabilitation. Andover, Boston

Maddison P J, Isenberg D A, Woo P, Glass D M (eds) Oxford textbook of rheumatology, 2nd edn, vol. 2. Oxford University Press, Oxford

Murtagh J 1994 General practice. McGraw-Hill, New South Wales

Chronic back and neck pain

Panzer R J, Black E R, Griner P F (eds) 1991 Diagnostic strategies for common medical problems. American College of Physicians, Philadelphia

Souhami R L, Moxham J (eds) 1994 Textbook of medicine. Churchill Livingstone, Edinburgh

Swash M (ed) 1994 Hutchison's clinical methods. W B Saunders, London

Urinary tract problems

Homma Y, Imajo C, Takahashi S, Kawabe K, Aso Y 1994 Urinary symptoms and urodynamics in a normal elderly population. Scandinavian Journal of Urology and Nephrology (Supplement) 157: 27–30

Epilepsy

Allen C M C, Lueck C J 2003 Diseases of the nervous system. In Haslett C, Chilvers E R, Hunter J A A, Boon N A (eds) Davidson's principles and practice of medicine, 19th edn. Churchill Livingstone, Edinburgh

Fry J, Sandler G 1993 Common diseases. Their nature, presentation and care, 5th edn. Kluwer Academic, London

Scadding J W, Gibbs J 2002 Neurological disease. In Souhami R L, Moxham J (eds). Textbook of medicine, 4th edn. Churchill Livingstone, Edinburgh

Migraine and other causes of recurrent headache

Classification Committee of the International Headache Society 1988 Classification and diagnostic criteria for headache disorders, cranial neuralgias and facial pain. Cephalgia 8(suppl. 7): 1–96

Goadsby P J, Olesen J 1996 Fortnightly review: diagnosis and management of migraine. British Medical Journal 312: 1279–1283

Common gastrointestinal disorders

Apley J, MacKeith R 1968 The child and his symptoms: a comprehensive approach. Blackwell Scientific, Oxford

Harris A, Misiewicz J J 2001 ABC of the upper gastro intestinal tract: management of *helicobactor pylori* infection. British Medical Journal 323: 1047–1050

Jones R, Goeting N (eds) 1992 Current approaches: Current gastroenterology topics in general practice. Duphar Laboratories,

Levenstein S 1998 Stress and peptic ulcer: life beyond helicobactor. British Medical Journal 316: 538–541

Logan R P H, Walker M M 2001 ABC of the upper gastro intestinal tract: epidemiology and diagnosis of *Helicobactor pylori* infection. British Medical Journal 323: 920–922

Misiewicz J J, Pounder R E, Venables C W (eds) 1994 Diseases of the gut and pancreas, 2nd edn. Blackwell Scientific, Oxford

Prescribing/medicines utilisation

House of Commons Health Committee 1994 Second report. Priority setting in the NHS: the NHS drugs budget. Minutes of evidence and appendices, vol. II. HMSO, London

The primary–secondary care interface

Bailey J, Black M, Wilkin D 1994 Specialist outreach clinics in general practice. British Medical Journal 308: 1083–1086

Coulter A 1998 Managing demand at the interface between primary and secondary care. British Medical Journal 316: 1974–1976

Hodgkin K 1985 Towards earlier diagnosis. A guide to primary care. Churchill Livingstone, Edinburgh

Inglehart J K 1993 Managed care. New England Journal of Medicine 327: 742–747

NHS Management Executive 1991 Integrating primary and secondary care. Department of Health, London

Orton P 1994 Shared care. Lancet 344: 1413–1415

Rosleff F, Lister G 1995 European healthcare trends: towards managed care in Europe. Coopers & Lybrand, London

Starfield B 1992 Primary care: concept, evaluation and policy. Oxford University Press, Oxford

Wilkin D 1992 Patterns of referral: explaining variation. In Roland M, Coulter A (eds) Hospital referrals. Oxford University Press, Oxford

Community care

Atkinson J M 1999 Community Care. In: Porter M, Alder B, Abraham C (eds) Psychology and sociology applied to medicine. Churchill Livingstone, Edinburgh

NHS Management Executive 1991 Integrating primary and secondary care. Department of Health, London

Royal Commission on Long Term Care 1999 With respect to old age: long term care – rights and responsibilities. Stationery Office, London

Secretaries of State 1989 Caring for people. Community care in the next decade and beyond. HMSO, London

Secretary of State for Health 1997 The new NHS, modern, dependable. Department of Health, London

Secretary of State for Health 1999 Saving lives: our healthier nation. Department of Health, London

Complementary and alternative medicine

Assendelft W J J, Bouter L M, Knipschild P G 1996 Complications of spinal manipulation: a comprehensive review of the literature. Journal of Family Practice 42:475–480

Berliner H S 1985 A system of scientific medicine. Tavistock, New York

Erns E 2000 Herbal medicines: where is the evidence? BMJ 321: 395–396

Linde K, Clausius N, Ramirez G, et al 1997 Are the clinical effects of homoeopathy placebo effects? A meta-analysis of placebo-controlled trials. Lancet 350:834–843

Patel M, Gutzwiller F, Paccaud F, Marazzi A 1989 A meta-analysis of acupuncture for chronic pain. International Journal of Epidemiology 18(4):900–6

Genetics in primary care

Rose P, Lucassen A 1999 Practical genetics for primary care. Oxford University Press, Oxford

Research in primary care

Bradley C 1998 Qualitative vs quantitative research methods. In Carter Y (ed.) Research methods in primary care. Radcliffe Medical Press, Oxford

Department of Health 1993 Research for health. Department of Health, London

Haines A, Donald A 1998 Making better use of research findings. British Medical Journal 317: 72–75

Medical Research Council 1997 Primary health care. MRC, London

National Working Group on Research and Development in Primary Care 1997 Research and development in primary care. National Working Group Report. NHS Executive, Leeds

Smith LFP 1997 Research general practices: what, who and why? British Journal of General Practice 47: 83–86

Some useful medical websites

Please note that these website addresses were correct at time of going to press, but websites can be transitory.

Accident prevention	www.rospa.com/CMS/index.asp	Royal Society for the Prevention of Accidents
Acupuncture	www.medical-acupuncture.co.uk	British Medical Acupuncture Society
Addictions	www.addictionresourceguide.com	Resources guide
AIDS	www.medfash.org.uk	Medical Foundation for AIDS and Sexual Health
Alcohol abuse	www.alcoholconcern.org.uk	Resources guide
Alternative Medicine	www.healthy.net/CLINIC/therapy/index.asp	
Arthritis	www.arthritis.org	Rheumatoid Arthritis Foundation
Asthma	www.gpiag-asthma.org	General Practice Airways Group
Bedwetting	www.enuresis.org.uk	
Blindness	www.rnib.org	Royal National Institute for the Blind
British Medical Journal	www.bmj.com	
Bullying	www.successunlimited.co.uk/trauma.htm	
Cancer	www.cancernews.com	
Child abuse	www.yesican.org	
Choking	www.dhce.liv.ac.uk/clinicalskills/6/choking/sld004.htm	Liverpool University – how to save someone from choking using Heimlich's manoeuvre
Constipation	www.emedicine.com/ereg/topic111	
Contraception	www.merck.com/pubs/mmanual-home/ch241/htm	Merck Manual
Counselling	www.counselling.co.uk	British Association for Counselling
Deafness	www.rnid.org	Royal National Institute for Deaf People
Death	www.bbc.co.uk/education/archive/grave/index.shtml	What to do when someone dies
Defibrillators	www.resus.org.uk/pages/aed.htm	Guidelines for defibrillators
Dementia	www.ion.ucl.ac.uk	UK National Hospital for Neurology
Dental Health	www.dentalhealth.org.uk/tellme	British Dental Foundation
Department of Health	www.doh.gov.uk	Access to UK Departments of Health
Diabetes	www.diabetes.org.uk	Diabetes UK
Diet and nutrition	www.bda.com	British Dietetic Association
	www.nutrition.org.uk	British Nutrition Foundation
Epilepsy	www.epilepsy.org.uk	British Epilepsy Association
Evidence based medicine	www.ebandolier.com	Bondolier website
	www.york.ac.uk/inst/crd	NHS Centre for reviews & Dissemination
Food poisoning	www.digestivedisorders.org.uk/leaflets/foodpoi.html	
Fungal infections	www.leeds.ac.uk/mbiology/ug/dental/dfungi.htm	
General Medical Council	www.gmc-uk.org.uk	
General Practice	www.internet-gp.com/gpsites	List of GP websites
Genetic counselling	www.uclan.ac.uk/facs/ethics/gencoun.htm	Ethics of Heart Disease
	www.cafamily.org.uk	Family Heart Association
	www.pccs.org.uk/index.html	Primary Care Cardiovascular Society
HMSO	www.hmso.gov.uk	UK government publications
House dust mite	www.user.globalnet.co.uk/~aair/mites-htm	
Impotence (erectile dysfunction)	www.informed.org.uk/	
Infertility	www.child.org.uk	UK National Infertility Support Network
Influenza	www.phls.co.uk/facts/influenza/flu.htm	Public Health Laboratory Service
Insomnia	www.londonhealth.co.uk/insomnia.asp	
Literature searching	www.ncbi.nim.nih.gov/PubMed	Free access to Medline
	www.nelh-pc.nhs.uk	Primary care branch of NHS library
	www.omni.ac.uk	UK medical subject listing
Meningitis	www.medinfo.co.uk/conditions/meningitis.html	
Menopause	www.the-bms.org	British Menopause Society

Mental Health	www.warne.ox.ac.uk/cebmh	MIND website
Migraine	www.migraine.org.uk/800frame.htm	UK Migraine Association
MMR vaccination	www.doh.gov.uk/mmrvac.htm	Mumps, measles and rubella vaccine
National Health Service (UK)	www.nhsia.nhs.uk	NHS portal site
NICE	www.nice.org.uk	UK National Institute for Clinical Excellence
Obesity	www.aso.org.uk	Association for the Study of Obesity
NHS Scotland	www.show.scot.nhs.uk	Scottish Health on the Web (SHOW)
Prescription Medicines	www.fda.gov	USA Food & Drug Administration
	www.open.gov.uk/mca	UK Medicines Control Agency
PRODIGY	www.prodigy.nhs.uk	Prescribing guidance for UK GPs
Prostatic Disease	www.prostatitis.org	
Royal College of General Practitioners	www.rcgp.org.uk	
Self help groups	www.patient.co.uk/selfhelp	
Sexually transmitted diseases	www.shastd.org.uk	
Skin diseases	www.telemedicine.org/stanford.htm	
	Tray.dermatology.uiowa.edu	
Smoking cessation	www.ash.org.uk	Action on Smoking and health (ASH)
Sports medicine	www.nsmi.org.uk	UK National Sports Medicine Institute
Stroke	www.stroke.org.uk	The UK Stroke Association
Travel advice	www.fco.gov.uk	UK Foreign & Commonwealth Office
	www.traveldoctor.co.uk/info.htm	
Verrucae(warts)	www.feetforlife.org/verrucae.htm	Society of Chiropodists
World Health Organisation	www.who.int	

More general useful websites

www.bbc.co.uk/health/ask_doctor/nrt Health and fitness with on-line doctors to answer queries

www.icircle.co.uk Specialises in women's problems

www.nhsdirect.nhs.uk An NHS site aimed at providing guidance on whether to contact a doctor

www.irishhealth.com Health information divided into categories on, for example, children's health, skin conditions and sexual health

www.mca.gov.uk Website for the Medicines Control Agency

www.show.scot.nhs.uk Online health information provided by NHS Scotland

www.surgerydoor.co.uk An excellent site with information on everything from alternative medicine to travel advice. Instant access to the Cochrane Library, journals and even Harrison's 'Textbook of internal medicine'

www.patient.org.uk A directory of websites providing information on health, disease and illness

www.chic.org.uk Produced by the Consumer Health Information Centre for the consumer

Index